Erika Sutter
Seen with Other Eyes

LIVES
LEGACIES
LEGENDS

Left:
Gertrud Stiehle

Right:
Erika Sutter

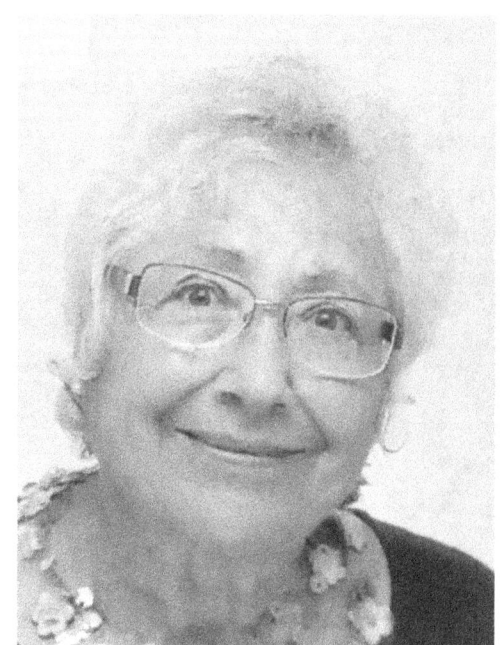
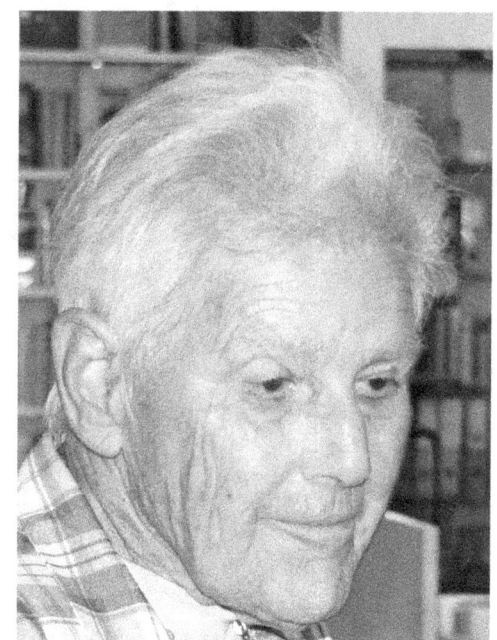

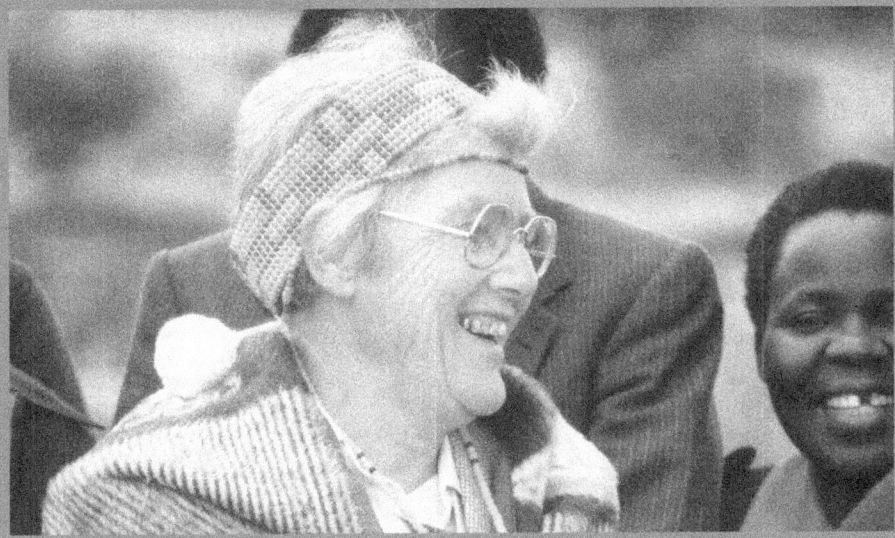

Erika Sutter
Seen with Other Eyes
Memories of a Swiss Eye Doctor in Rural South Africa

Told by Gertrud Stiehle

With a foreword by Mamphela Ramphele
and a preface and one chapter by Frances Lund

Basel
Basler Afrika Bibliographien
2013

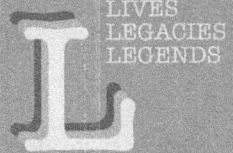

Kindly supported by DM Echange et Mission, Lausanne; Mission 21, Basel; Südafrika Mission Trägerverein; Basler Mission Trägerverein; Bertha Hess Cohn-Stiftung Basel; and a number of generous individuals.

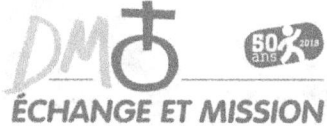

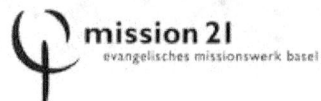

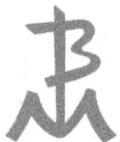

© The authors
© The photographers
© Basler Afrika Bibliographien
PO Box 2037
CH-4001 Basel
Switzerland
www.baslerafrika.ch

All rights reserved.
Originally published in 2011 as "Erika Sutter: Mit anderen Augen gesehen. Erinnerungen einer Schweizer Augenärztin".
Translated by Anu Lannen, Basel; edited by J. M. Jenkins, Basel.

Cover photo: Erika Sutter at her farewell from the Venda Care Groups, 1984. Private Collection Erika Sutter

ISBN 978-3-905758-33-7

ISSN 1660-9638

Contents

A healer and torch bearer
A foreword: Mamphela Ramphele VII

Preface by Frances Lund VIII

In lieu of an introduction:
Immersing myself in the life of Erika Sutter 1

| I | **The Roots** | 3 |

II	**Childhood and Adolescence**	6
	A happy time: Early childhood years in Basel and holidays in Valais	6
	Paradise was in Troistorrents	7
	The youngest	9
	School days	9
	A conflict-laden adolescence	11

III	**University Studies during World War II and starting in a profession**	13
	The challenge of choosing a career	13
	Studying during turbulent times	14
	Not quite as planned: the start of professional life	16
	Two unmarried daughters set up house on the Spalenberg	18
	Life during the Second World War	20

IV	**Preparing for Africa**	25
	First contact with the mission	25
	A circuitous route leads to a successful plunge	25
	Two happy years in Sweden	26
	A decision, and a second contact with the mission	28
	Final preparations and departure	29

V	**The Path to Ophthalmology**	32
	Settling down in Elim	32
	The laboratory – a long working day	37
	Nationalisation of the schools: the spread of "Bantu Education"	39
	A new challenge: Medical School in Johannesburg	40
	The year of residency	46
	Specializing in ophthalmology	47

VI	**Head of the Eye Hospital in Elim**	50
	Returning to Elim as a doctor	50
	Her own home with a garden	52

	Making music in the mission setting	56
	Vacation and more training	56
	Language – understanding – communication	57
	Stories about spectacles	59
	Apartheid and forced resettlement	60
	Apartheid and Christianity	63
	Working and living in South Africa under apartheid	66
	New possibilities open up: a second ophthalmologist in Elim	68
	The School for the Diploma in Ophthalmic Nursing	69
	The Eye Doctor's own eye problems	76

VII The most meaningful years in Erika's life: The Care Groups
(written by Frances Lund) — 78

Community eye health – the development of the Care Groups	78
Leadership and being a leader	81
Health education based on what people know	82
Managing time and people	83
Finding support	85
Voluntary work	86
The Care Groups and the church	86
The repressive political environment	88
Ubuntu: People are a gold mine	89

VIII Retirement and the return to Basel — 94

Preparations for retirement	94
The grand departure from Elim	95
The return to Basel, and new contacts	97
Passing on knowledge and experience	98
Experiences with apartheid, seen from afar – and the beginning of change	99
New horizons	100
Honours	104
Drawing strength from family	106
Limited time, and thoughts of death	107

IX A final look back and forward — 111

A conversation between Erika Sutter and Gertrud Stiehle	111

Illustrations — 122

Bibliography — 123

List of publications by Erika Sutter	123
Further publications on the Care Groups	124

A healer and torch bearer
A foreword

My first encounter with Erika Sutter was in 1978. What could have been an impersonal relationship between an eye specialist and an inexperienced young doctor was transformed into a strong warm personal friendship by her generosity.

It was the remote encounter through a reference of a toddler with a damaged eye after a bout of measles to the famous eye doctor in Elim Hospital that Erika used to introduce herself to me as a consummate compassionate doctor. I was then a young inexperienced doctor banished to Lenyenye Township in Tzaneen, Limpopo Province. Dr Sutter not only attended to the child I referred to her, but she recognised my ignorance about the cause of the problem and wrote me a detailed report about the vitamin A deficiency that was responsible for the condition that destroyed the child's eye. It was a lesson I never forgot and it helped me to help the community in the Lenyenye area to take preventive action by feeding their children vitamin rich food and vegetables such as carrots and pumpkins.

Erika followed this encounter with a visit to my home and to Ithusheng Community Health Centre in Lenyenye. Her gentle kind eyes and smile made me feel connected immediately. She shared her Care Group work experiences with me and that helped shape our own Community Health Worker Program as Ithusheng in the Tzaneen area. This model continues still across the country, where Mankuba Ramalepe, a former senior nurse at Ithusheng, continues to inspire communities to help themselves.

Erika is one of a kind. She embodies the values of a consistent feminine leadership style that emphasises flexibility, humility, diversity of opinion and service. She not only used her expertise to help those in need of health care but used the power of knowledge to promote feminine style leadership in the communities she worked with. She sought to transform the missionary society and medical profession she was part of from male dominance notions of power into accepting the power of a feminine style of leadership. Her transformative approach was through influence and the power of example. She has touched lives that changed radically for the better through her enabling leadership approach.

Erika is also remarkable in how she exemplifies a life lived to the full. She has not only given a lot of herself, her youth and her expertise, but has remained fully alive to the joys of life. Her home in Basel is an oasis of beauty and charm. Modest but wonderfully decorated with memories of her journey in life. Above all, her smile and love of life and people shines through her kind eyes always. She is the embodiment of how life should be lived in service of humanity and in living out the best in oneself.

I am richer as a person for having encountered this remarkable woman as a colleague, a mentor, a friend and a fellow global citizen. She is a torch bearer who not only opened the physical eyes of those she encountered but also their spiritual eyes to appreciate the power they had within them. She is a true healer of minds and souls. We have much to thank her for.

Mamphela Ramphele

Preface

I met Erika Sutter for the first time in the mid-1980s. I was doing a Master's degree, and chose the Elim Care Groups as one of three South African case studies in primary health care. Our friendship developed over the years. I met many members of her family, and was able to visit her on her seventieth, eightieth and ninetieth birthdays in Basel. I was included in her remarkable circle of friends, many of them involved in support work with the Basel-based anti-apartheid movement. In Durban, my friend Davine and I were graced with visits to our home of some of these friends from Switzerland.

Erika has written extensively about her medical and community work in rural South Africa, mobilising women in Care Groups to address the problem of trachoma. In her academic and popular writings as an "eye doctor", she has consistently emphasised the role of others. Her main purpose has been that others could learn from and replicate the knowledge developed by Care Group members themselves. She also wanted the role of South African and international colleagues, and in particular that of Selina Maphorogo, leader of the Care Groups, to be recognised.

Her books and articles were on the reading list of the course I taught for a Master's degree in Social Policy at the University of KwaZulu-Natal (then, University of Natal). The students learned about the specific approach of the Care Groups to community mobilisation, and about the benefits of a preventive rather than a curative approach to health care. Our international student group, from countries in sub-Saharan Africa, Europe and the Americas, frequently approached me after reading her work. They would say: "The reading material is interesting, but who was she really? What motivated *her*? Where did she come from? What gave her the idea of doing this work, and how did she sustain the work and herself?"

Their questions point to a problem at the heart of how people learn about community development, social policy and social change. Pioneers such as Erika who break new ground tend to be coy and silent about their own role, whether they are constrained by modesty, religion, or other factors. Perhaps this is also something that women in particular tend to do. Whatever the reason, it means that a crucial factor in development of the projects remains hidden: who the leaders are, what influenced their choice of career, and why they did what they did. A person such as Erika, in the health field, is a medical doctor. In developing the Care Groups, she puts her acquired medical status on the line. She has to learn to change her own thinking and practice. She has to allow complexity and contradiction rather than diagnostic certainty. She has to listen very carefully to local explanations of where disease comes from and how it spreads. She has to acknowledge that there is no "perfect plan", but an organic and flexible process of development.

In mid 2007 I was visiting in Basel and Erika showed me her most recent book, *The Community is my University*, on which she worked with Selina. In that book, Erika provided an opportunity to highlight Selina's central role as a health educator and community mobiliser. I said: "Erika, this is a beautiful and useful production. You have given Selina a platform. Now what about your story?" Erika then said that she would never write this, as amongst other things, it was "too personal".

A few months later she phoned me at Christmas time. She said that she had been talking to her dear friend Gertud Stiehle, and was reconsidering writing a more personal book. In January 2008 I wrote in response:

Now, about what I was meaning when we spoke about why you should write your own story. I have long thought, there is such a contradiction … Many of the very good people [in development work] are those who are really altruistic. Part of that altruism is that they do not put their own 'agency' forward – they do not tell us what really drives them personally. It could be God, but I am getting at something behind or alongside God as well. Some of it comes from childhood experiences, but we cannot learn from these, because the good people think they should not talk about themselves.

[...] I consider that you are a very, very interesting person, and many people outside your family would be interested in how you grew up, how you were with your siblings, boy friends and girl friends, at school, at church, at play; who you were in love with (not only your dog Mambuxu ...) and the decision to go into the mission and your profession. As time goes by, people will want to know more about the Care Groups, and Elim, but there is a missing part of the big picture, as far as I know, and that is you. You have given Selina so much space to tell her story. You have a story too.

Erika needed someone who would, as she put it, help her to let her memories flow. And her friend Gertrud Stiehle was the only person she could imagine playing this role. Gertrud had become an anthropologist/ethnographer in her late sixties, doing an intriguing and sensitive study of widows in the Cameroon, allowing insights into their complex situation – powerful as well as powerless, oppressed but also agents of change.

In this present book, Erika, now in her nineties, allows herself, her history, her life and loves, her interests and motivations to come to the surface. She is one of the last of the Swiss South Africa Mission fraternal workers to have stayed for so long in South Africa. Her narrative starts in Switzerland. Then, in South Africa, it spans the worst of the apartheid period. When she retired to Switzerland, she was active in the anti-apartheid movement before the transition to democracy in 1994. In creating this book, she has confronted her past, some of which has become visible to her for the first time.

In the present, Erika, Gertrud, and to a lesser extent myself, have had to wrestle with, and negotiate about, what became an enormous and complex undertaking. For me personally, the collaboration with these remarkable and brave women of Basel has enabled me to think about my own future in more confident and creative ways. My friendship with Erika and Gertrud has been loving, inspiring, and liberating and filled with laughter – a gracious and graced gift.

Frances Lund,
Associate Professor in the School of Built Environment and Development Studies, University of Kwazulu-Natal

In lieu of an introduction:

Immersing myself in the life of Erika Sutter

"Come in!" Erika Sutter opens the door to her flat on the top floor of a modern four-storey building in the Bachletten neighbourhood of Basel. She's become smaller with age, and rather bent, but despite her ninety-three years she scurries agilely in front of me into the corridor. I admire her shining white hair and her lavender-blue sweater, which flatters the porcelain complexion of her well-balanced features. Arriving in the living room, she turns and looks up at me attentively with eyes that often appear faintly red-rimmed.

Erika has been my friend and companion on a joint project that has stretched over three years, with interruptions due to trips, illnesses, hospital stays, or breaks that were simply necessary. Each week she shared a piece of her life story with me, and I created the German original of the present book, using dozens of audio recordings, letters, other documents, and information from people who know Erika and her story.

I've scarcely had time to slip on my now-accustomed pair of house shoes when Erika calls out, "Just look at the blue cranesbill in bloom!" and opens the door to the balcony that faces East. The view extends over and beyond the old trees of Basel's zoological gardens, into the vast overcast sky, and across the hill called the Gempenstollen. Nearby, the eye comes to rest on Basel's main railway station. Like snakes – some silvery and some dark – international trains arrive and depart, contributing to the wonderful sea of lights at night.

Thriving here on the balcony in large plant troughs are lovingly collected wild plants – some given by friends – from Swiss regions like the Hinterrhein and the Jura. They share space with rose bushes, bamboo, the sprawling and delicate richly coloured blossoms of yellow crown vetch, clematis, Cape fuchsia, grasses, lavender, ever-fruiting strawberries, blueberries, seasonal plants, and herbs that Erika dries and grinds to powder. At the far end of the long balcony sits a small greenhouse. Pottering around in the roof garden is Erika's great joy, and she's been relieved of the most difficult work thanks to an automatic irrigation system and the occasional help of a gardener from the senior citizens' support organisation Pro Senectute.

Let us turn our attention quickly to Erika's "miracle plant", the one she has a very special relationship with: *Oenothera odorata*, the fragrant evening primrose. The plant's large, bright yellow blossoms give off a delicate fragrance, blooming for one night only. It grows on the other side of the flat, on the balcony that faces West, amongst grasses, heather, harebells, and other plants that enjoy the conditions there. From this balcony we look out over the rooftops to France, to the hills of Sundgau. With a little luck, Erika can spot a friend on one of the balconies two blocks away and wave "hello". She's at home in this neighbourhood.

Much like the botanical microcosm on her balconies, the interior of Erika's flat displays her own life in miniature. In both of her sunny rooms and the corridor mementos from Africa catch the eye: colourful bands of beadwork, and objects decorated with beads; blankets and pillowcases made of African fabrics; a carved stick like a snake; mahogany carvings, and woven wall hangings – including my favourite piece, a tapestry depicting a tree with weaver birds' nests. Interspersed between them are a Rothko print, a spinet, some nice old pieces of family furniture, books and more books, a record collection, and the blue-flowering South African hanging plant *Streptocarpus*.

Erika's ease with the aids and appliances of old age is especially impressive: elevator, electric bed, armchair, computer workstation, magnifying glasses, hearing aid, cane – and, not to be forgotten, an alarm device worn on her wrist in case of emergencies. Her cabinets and drawers are organised so everything is easy to find. When I mistakenly disrupt the strict military order of her cutlery box while putting things away, she quickly explains why things must be arranged just so and not otherwise. Still, there are days when I enter the flat and see things lying about, a sign of how Erika can quickly tire and isn't always able to keep up with her ambitious workload the way she once did. She is very grateful for the support of her dear neighbour Annegreth as well as that of Izeta from Bosnia, who has helped her in the household for years.

Erika sits across from me at her round table. Twenty years separate us. A mutual interest in conjuring up her life's memories, and capturing those she wishes to pass on, connects us. Today we'll begin with her roots. Where does she come from?

Gertrud Stiehle

Gertrud and Erika working on the book, 2010

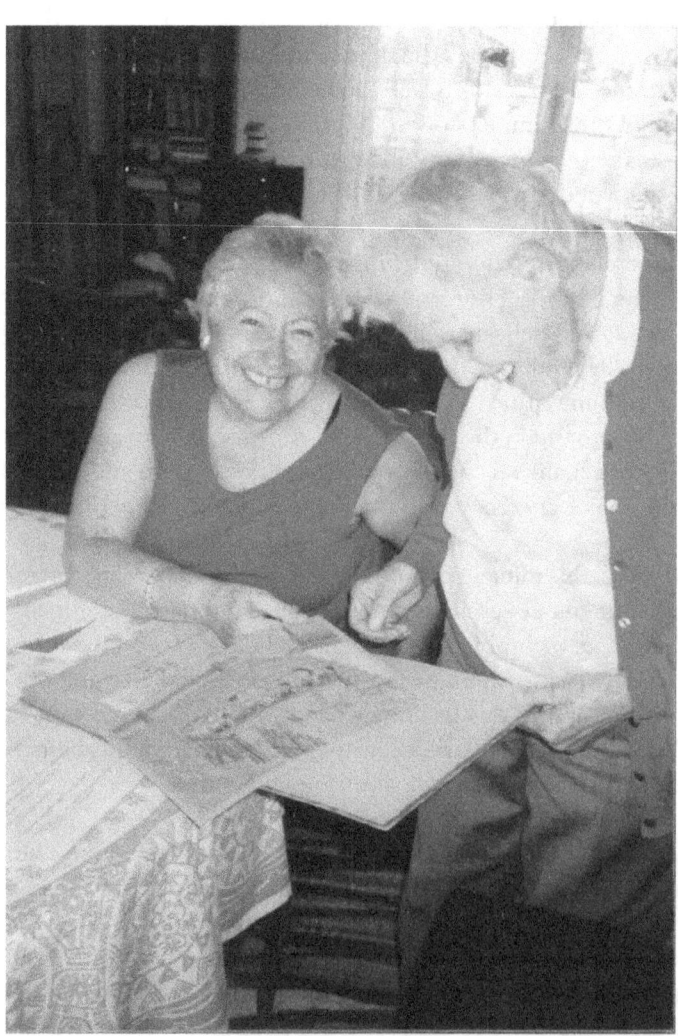

I The Roots

Erika remembers:

> I know a lot more about my father's side of the family, since he enjoyed telling us about the family much more than my mother did. My great-grandfather, Johann Jakob Sutter (1812–1865), came from Bühler in Appenzell-Ausserrhoden. He was the youngest of ten children and lost his mother early on. Thanks solely to the help of an older brother, he acquired some knowledge and skills beyond his rudimentary school education, enabling him to found a small embroidery business. He became interested in politics early in life, becoming a lay magistrate when he was only twenty-five, and eventually the President of the Canton *(Landammann)* and a member of the Swiss Parliament – positions that demanded big investments of time and money. In his home there was always just enough to get by on. Of his eleven children, six survived childhood. There's a story in our family about the unusual way he taught his sons to swim. There was a small waterfall in Bühler that emptied into a large pool of water. My great-grandfather would stand at the top of the waterfall and toss his boys in, one after the other!
>
> When it came to the youngest son, my grandfather Karl Theodor Sutter, there was no money left to finance further education. So he was sent away to make his own fortune. He wound up in Genoa and was hired as a deckhand on a ship bound for Alexandria. There he landed an apprenticeship in a cotton factory and eventually worked his way up to a good position. Once he had "made something of himself", he returned to Bühler to fetch his wife-to-be, Emma Fisch, my grandmother. She was a delicate, beautiful woman, whom I sadly only know from photos. They had two children, first Ernst Theodor, my father, and then Ida.

Erika's father, Ernst Theodor Sutter, was born in 1881 in Alexandria. He attended a German school there, acquiring a very correct High German, which he then had to unlearn thoroughly when, at the age of fourteen, he was sent to Switzerland to attend the Cantonal High School in St. Gallen, where he had to learn the dialect of German spoken in that part of Switzerland.

> He lived on his own in a single unheated room, where he had to break the ice in the jug each morning in order to wash himself. My father loved to recall his schoolboy pranks. There was also a story he told about the group of teetotallers at the High School. This was a new movement in those days. Back then, it was still common to give children wine to drink at St. Gallen's annual children's festival, as there was nothing else on offer. So this group of students set up a stand serving soft drinks, and from then on wine was no longer given to the children. My father remained a total abstainer for the rest of his life.

Following his confirmation in the Reformed Church, Erika's father became interested in the ideas of the Enlightenment and soon after declared himself to be an agnostic. He studied chemistry in Zürich and also for a year in Berlin. However, in Berlin, lectures on ancient languages and Middle High German captured his attention even more than chemistry, for he had linguistic and literary interests in addition to his scientific pursuits. Erika still remembers the classical quotations and many stories that her father told and read to her and her siblings.

Erika's father met his future wife, Meta Ris, at a formal dance in Zürich, where she was training as a teacher. They married shortly after she had qualified, and moved to Mannheim in Germany, where Erika's father started his first job with the pharmaceutical company Boehringer. The eldest of the four Sutter children, Hans and Trudi, were born there. Later the family moved to Basel when Erika's father got a job as chemist at Ciba. He remained there until his retirement. It was in Basel that Ernst and Erika were born, the second brother-and-sister pair.

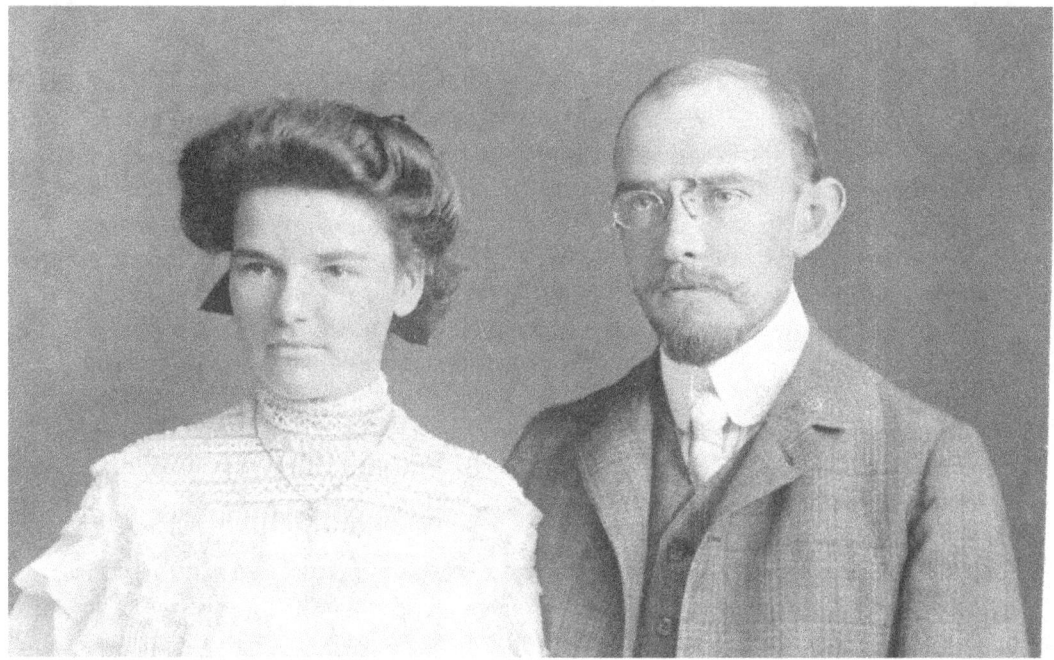

Meta and Theodor Sutter-Ris, Erika's parents, as a newly married couple, August 1905

Erika describes her Auntie Ida, her father's younger sister by two years, with admiration and affection, as a special person who played an important role in Erika's life and that of the entire family:

> Much like her brother, Auntie Ida became an agnostic early in life, and even refused to be confirmed as a member of the church, which was unusual in 1898. And the fact that she, as a woman, studied botany at the ETH (Federal Polytechnic) in Zürich was practically a sensation! She married a fellow student, Otto Schüep, who became Professor of Plant Morphology in the University of Basel The family lived in Reinach, Baselland, and were the only close relatives with whom we maintained strong ties.

Erika's roots on her mother's side lie in the Canton of Bern. Her great-grandfather, Friedrich Ris (1806–87) was a secondary school teacher of classical languages and religion in Burgdorf, and later became an associate professor of philosophy at the University of Bern. On account of his Enlightenment ideas, Ris was attacked vehemently in several writings by the renowned Swiss novelist, the pastor Jeremias Gotthelf. In *Zeitgeist und Bernergeist* (The Spirit of the Times and the Bernese Spirit), for example, Gotthelf declares, "We can gain nothing from *'Riesen'* (giants) and other monsters and unbelievers." (This is a play on the name "Ris", which sounds almost the same as the German word for giant, Riese). In the same text, Gotthelf dubs Ris, *"the inventor of the Riesenreligion* (i.e. gigantic religion)". Elsewhere, in his *Briefen* (Letters), the author writes: "I was not impressed by Ris, I considered that he was pretentious." According to an account found in one of his granddaughter's letters, Friedrich Ris eventually retired early and spent his days silently pondering at his desk.

Friedrich Ris's first son, Theodor, became a doctor in Thun and later in Sigriswil. His younger son Moritz, Erika's grandfather, wanted to become a doctor as well, but was compelled to go into training in a business firm. He worked as an accountant in Winterthur, but eventually he dared to break out, and went to Silesia *(Schlesien)*, where he completed an apprenticeship as a gardener, which he found very satisfying. He eventually went to Goldswil, near Interlaken, in the mountain area near Bern *(Berner Oberland)*, where he lived to the end of his days. He taught himself about homoeopathy and the use of medicinal herbs, and thanks to his detailed knowledge he became known throughout the *Berner Oberland* as a healer and naturopath.

Erika doesn't have any direct memories of this grandfather. Her mother wrote a very affectionate account of his life, and was evidently very fond of him, although he was a taciturn, unhappy man who was by turns withdrawn and quick-tempered, so that his family was almost afraid of him. Music meant a lot to him. He used to sit by himself quietly playing the concert zither – yet another self-taught skill.

Moritz Ris married a Jewish Christian, Nathalie Loebell from Stettin, a beautiful but mentally ill woman who – Erika believes – suffered from depression. She eventually went blind – did she suffer from glaucoma, like Erika? Her two daughters, Meta, Erika's mother, and Helene, grew up mostly in the care of relatives, since their mother was ill so often and their father scarcely looked after them. Reading about her grandfather in her mother's memoirs, Erika grows thoughtful:

> I probably inherited more from my grandparents on my mother's side than I used to think. My grandfather had the same love of nature, plants, and medicine that runs like a thread through my own life. I also studied biology and medicine, of course. And I also share his fondness for music. And could I have inherited a predisposition for depression from my grandmother Loebell?

Erika's mother Meta, née Ris (1881–1961), suffered for years from the lack of family warmth and affection in her childhood. She did not have a good relationship with her only sister Helene, two years her junior, as Erika's mother always felt neglected in comparison with her younger sister. Though Helene was Erika's godmother, they eventually lost all contact with her.

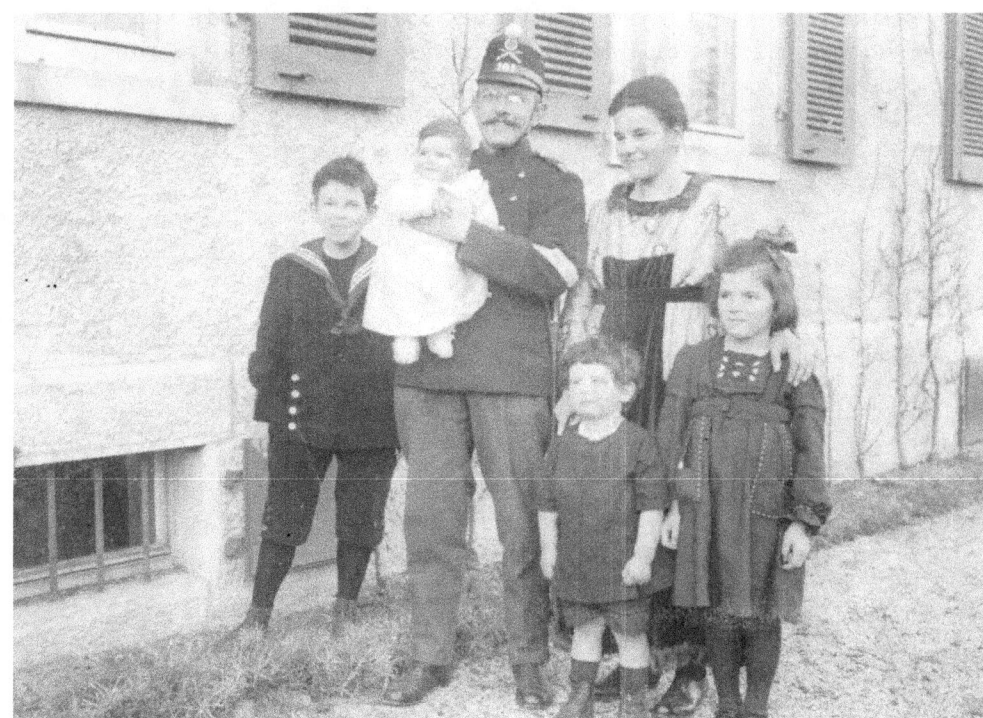

The Sutter family on the day of Erika's baptism, 1918

II Childhood and Adolescence

A happy time: Early childhood years in Basel and holidays in Valais

Erika Sutter was born in Basel on June 14th 1917, the youngest of four siblings. She comments that in an exemplary way her parents did exactly what she herself recommended in South Africa; they practised "family spacing" – not having children too close together. There were two pairs of Sutter children, with an interval of five years between them: Hans (1906) and Trudi (1909), born in Mannheim, and Ernst (1914) and Erika (1917), born in Basel. In those days, a middle-class family like Erika's could afford to hire someone to help out in the home. Lydia Bitzer also helped to look after the children, and she became an important figure in their lives. She used to sing with them, and she told them their first Bible stories, which they never would have heard at home otherwise.

Erika only has faint childhood memories of her older brother Hans, since he attended a boarding school and was away much of the time. By contrast, her older sister by eight years, Trudi, became her lifelong confidante. She was Erika's guide, role model, and eventually a substitute for their mother, who was often sick. Ernst, Erika's older brother by three years, was her favourite playmate. She conjures up a very early memory of him:

> At home we had an old Singer sewing machine that had a wooden cover. We'd sit together in it, as if we were in a boat, and pretend to paddle through the room. We must have been fairly little at the time to fit into that cover at all! Another time – I was probably four years old – Ernst and I were quite seriously ill at the same time and had to stay in bed. Someone read us a wonderful story. I wanted so much to read the story myself, that I took hold of the book and began reading it aloud almost effortlessly. As the youngest, I had learned the alphabet from my siblings early on. I was later told that Trudi was late to school that day, because everyone stood around and listened with astonishment as I read, even though I'd never been taught. Nevertheless, I didn't turn out to be a child prodigy.

Erika's mother with her four children in Goldswil, 1919. In front, from right to left: Ernst, Erika, Trudi, at the back, Hans

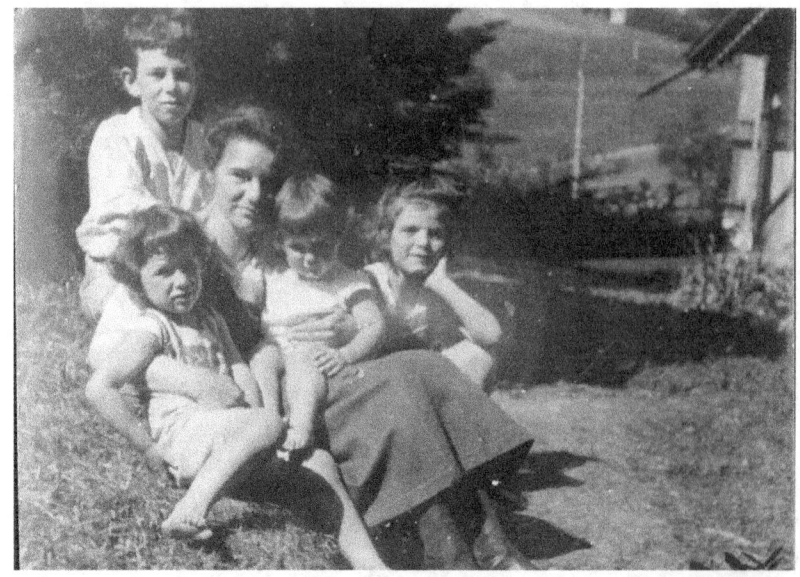

Paradise was in Troistorrents

On the whole, Erika enjoyed a carefree childhood in Basel and the family's vacation home in Troistorrents, in Valais. When she was four, her father was transferred to the Ciba factory in Monthey, Valais, and for the next eight years the Christmas holidays were the only time he lived with the family in Basel. Instead, the children went with their mother every year to spend their long summer vacations in Troistorrents, above Monthey, where they lived in the *Chalet Étoile* while the owner, the farmer Monsieur Dubosson, spent the summer living further up the mountain in Morgins, where the livestock were kept for the summer on the high pastures.

For the children it was nothing short of paradise; a glorious time of carefree play. In the sand at the foot of the chalet, Ernst and Erika built entire landscapes replete with villages, valleys, and bridges. And they also played at hospitals! After falling ill with intestinal tuberculosis when he was ten, and spending time in a sanatorium in Davos, Ernst had had his heart set on becoming a doctor. So in their games of make believe, the children brought his future plans to life. Ernst, as the head physician, opened a hospital. Erika was either a nurse or the mother of a patient, and they attended to all the dolls as patients. But later in life, it was Erika – not Ernst – who became a doctor.

The haystack was another favourite place to play:

> When Monsieur Dubosson came down from Morgins to make hay, he would take me on his knee atop the haystack and read me a story from one of my picture books, and I would say "oui" and "non" alternately – evidently at the wrong times in most cases, since the other children used to laugh. When it got dark at night, we'd play hide-and-seek in the haystack, and it was always wonderful to hide while our father tried to find us. Once, Trudi was hiding in the hay when she suddenly squealed, "A mouse is running across my tummy!" Trudi was always up to something. At the end of the day, she would usually tell us a story that she invented herself, often about a handsome youth with a violin. It's little things like this that have stuck in my memory.

At weekends, Erika's father took the family walking in the mountains. Friends of the children or other guests would often join them. But there was a little problem with Erika; whenever they came out above the tree line and walked across the blooming Alpine meadows, Erika would scarcely budge. She didn't want to step on a single little flower – and there were so many! Was it an early sign of her future as a biologist?

Many wonderful experiences and episodes are captured in the "Troistorrents Book" that the four children put together for their parents around 1930. In her meticulous calligraphy, Trudi documented what the summer vacations had meant to them over the years. She put in her own thoughts and poems, and the experiences that her younger siblings wrote down for her. The stories are about singing with the lute; about enjoying the company of friends, relatives, and villagers; about celebrations and thunderstorms. And last but not least, stories about their four-legged friends, which could not be left alone in Basel, and came with them every summer. There were the cats – first "Böhnli", then "Rugeli", then "Muggi" – and "Guggi," the parakeet. The Troistorrents Book is a cherished family document to which Erika – nicknamed "Riggi" by the others – also contributed, drawing on her talents and passion for sketching, painting, and storytelling. For example, Erika wrote about the hut that she, Ernst, and their friend Ida built in the forest:

Ida, Riggi, and Ernst loved the beauty of the forest. Riggi liked to walk alone in the woods. She would sit and listen to the birds. Often, she would tell herself stories.

One day, the children came up with the idea of building a hut, and began looking for a secluded spot:

Soon they discovered a grove of trees, unlike any they'd ever seen. Everywhere they looked they saw moss, rare mushrooms, and dark fir trees. They named the place "Pitamo," after all the *Pilze* (mushrooms), *Tannen* (fir trees), and *Moos* (moss). Here they found a moss carpet, a flat-topped rock that made a bench, and a cave. It was the right place to build their hut.

Just before they finished the roof, it was time to go home. After several days of bad weather, in which they busied themselves with homework, they went back to continue building, but discovered that:

The beautiful roof had collapsed. Riggi said merrily, "Well, we'll just have to clean everything up." And so they did. Then they sat down, admired the barberry bush *(berberitz)*, and listened to the birds.

Two pages from the book "Our holiday home"; Erika's story, written by Trudi and illustrated by Erika

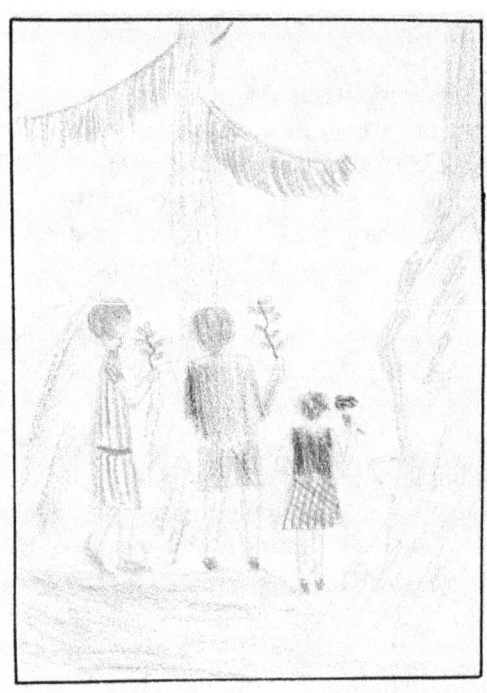

However, in the end, thanks to Ernst, who kept suggesting new ideas, they managed to build a roof over the rock bench, and then set about exploring the cave nearby:

Off went the three woodland children, clad in climbing boots and puttees, carrying sticks and candles. Ernst led the way, followed by Ida, with Riggi at the rear. There were no snakes to be found. But someone else had been in the cave – that was plain to see. They discovered a sort of altar at the back. They also found charred pieces of wood on the ground. The opening to the cave was just big enough to slip through. So it was here they held a housewarming. The fir tree in front of the rock bench was festooned with ivy and yellow oak branches. And the emblem for *"Pilz, Tanne, Moos"* was ceremoniously etched in the bark. Each child made a speech. This was followed by a torchlight procession through the Pitamo Grove. The cave and the altar were richly decorated. Ernst was made a priest and given the name Wodan. The two maidens were named Freya and Maya. The Pitamo Grove in Valais was transformed into a mysterious world of ancient Germanic myth.

The mountain air was particularly good for the two youngest children, Ernst and Erika, whose health was somewhat weak. Their family doctor in Basel prescribed them additional vacation time each year, for use between the official summer and autumn school holidays. Their father then gave Ernst Latin lessons in Troistorrents and, as a trained teacher, their mother was allowed to teach Erika primary school lessons beginning when she was six. In that way, they all managed to have an extended summer in the mountains

The youngest

How was it for Erika to be the youngest in the family? She lets out a little groan:

> Oh, like everyone else, I had to help out a lot in the household. As the youngest and the littlest, I had to do the dusting down low, and, whenever there was something missing at the dining table, I was sent to fetch it. It annoyed me a little, but that's just how it was! When we were washing the dishes together, we often sang rounds. Ernst thought I washed too slowly, so we switched roles. From then on, it was always my job to dry, and it remained that way for the rest of his life.

Contemplating the drawbacks of being the youngest, she suddenly began to laugh, realizing how she had succeeded in compensating for one childhood disadvantage:

> Every year at Christmas, our great-aunt Anna Fisch in Bühler in Appenzell sent us a package of the traditional decorated gingerbread cakes. My parents each got a big one; those for Hans, Trudi, and Ernst were progressively smaller, and mine was the smallest. Every year! That wasn't fair! Ernst was good at saving his gingerbread, and still had it long after I'd eaten mine. This bothered me so much that, to this day, whenever Basel's Autumn Fair comes around I buy myself a big, delicious piece of gingerbread and eat it all myself!

Were there no advantages in being the youngest?

> Certainly there were – for example, the fact that I learned to read so early, and learned many other things, simply by observing my older siblings, especially Trudi and Ernst.

School days

Erika's mother, who was a teacher, taught her at home for the first few years of primary school, but once she had reached the fourth class she went to school in the St. Johann schoolhouse near her home in Basel. Her memories of this period are faint: "It can't have been terribly dramatic, or I'd still remember it!" She only remembers an essay she was asked to write on the subject of "taking a walk." In it, she described how she enjoyed going for walks alone, just as she did in Troistorrents. The teacher praised the essay, and was also very impressed by the fact that she liked walking alone, which she considered unusual for a nine-year-old. Looking back, Erika wonders if the introversion and liking to be alone that she manifested early on might have been an early sign of her later feelings of depression.

At the end of the fourth class of primary school it was time for Erika to move to the girls' High School in Basel, the *Gymnasium am Kohlenberg*. Her sister Trudi had just finished the final class there and moved on to the Conservatory to study the violin. Trudi's class teacher had been Paul Gessler, and they had appreciated each other greatly, so she suggested to her parents that they should ask for Erika to be placed in his class. But it did not go well. Dr Gessler was expecting another Trudi; outgoing, animated, and clever. Instead, along came shy, introverted Erika. He was displeased with her, and she was so much afraid of him that when he took the class to Lörrach to learn swimming, Erika insisted that she could swim, so that she could join the swimmers in the deeper pools, and not stay with the non-swimmers under the teacher's eye. It was a bit of a risky decision on Erika's part:

> The highlight of our summers in Troistorrents was always a trip to Lake Geneva. Trudi had once given me a little swimming lesson in the shallow water. But swimming in a deep pool? I simply got in, held on to the edge, and gradually sensed that I could do it. From that point, I made rapid progress. In that same summer I jumped off a springboard into the river Rhine.

Left: Troistorrents 1922. Left to right: Erika, Hans, Ernst, Trudi Schüepp, Doris Amman, Trudi

Right: Trudi, Ernst, Erika; Lenzgasse, Basel, 1926

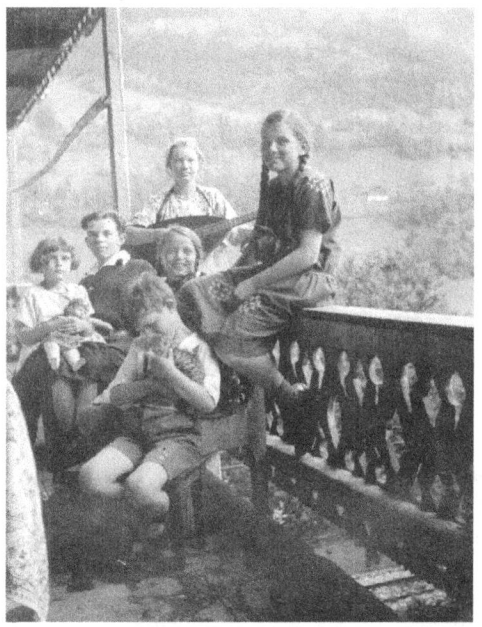
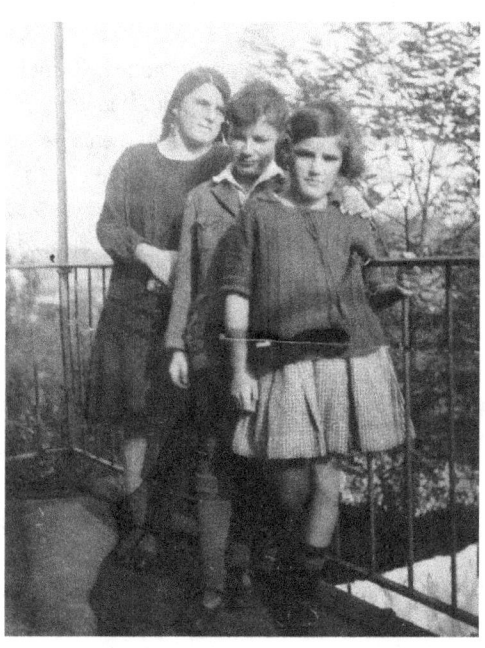

At the end of the second year of High School, the students had to opt for one of three types of course. They could simply continue until they had completed the twelfth year of schooling, and leave with a diploma. However, for University entrance it was necessary to have the more demanding school-leaving certificate called the *Matura*. Here there were two possibilities; a Federal *Matura* that was recognised in the whole country, and included Latin, and one which was administered by the Canton, which concentrated more on subjects like modern languages. With the Cantonal *Matura* students could study most subjects at the University – but not medicine. Dr Gessler advised Erika's parents that she should simply get the Diploma, saying, "The girl never really studies!" However, Erika's parents decide she should work for a *Matura* – but for the Cantonal one, because for the Federal examination she would have had to continue to suffer in Dr Gessler's class. Shy Erika submitted to her parents' wishes. She was not even thinking of studying medicine at that point. On the whole, the rest of her time in school went well, and she left with a Cantonal *Matura*.

After the final examinations, Erika's class went on a journey with the French teacher, Dr Roche. Erika enjoyed fourteen wonderful days, especially the unforgettable moment when, after an overnight train ride, she saw Venice for the first time, rising out of the sea in the early morning sunlight. And she encountered Italian art with amazement.

On the way home at the end of the trip, however, she suddenly realised that the first chapter of her life was coming to a close. She was overcome with a paralysing fear that she would not be able to cope with what lay ahead. Today, she attributes this intense experience to a depressing prediction made by her mother's best friend – which her mother reported to her. The friend had said, "Erika won't amount to anything! People who have difficulties at home will have them in life as well." This fatal judgment hit Erika hard at a time in her school career when she was already grappling with persistent feelings of depression, and it completely crushed her self-esteem.

A conflict-laden adolescence

Outwardly, Erika's school years were calm. But her inner development in adolescence was anything but peaceful. The usual conflicts involved in breaking away from home and family were intensified in her case into an almost pathological vicious circle. Nevertheless, although Erika was the member of the family who suffered most severely from problems with her relationship with her mother, she did eventually succeed, in retrospect, in understanding and forgiving her:

> Because of her own mother's illness, my mother spent years staying with other relatives and missed out on living in a family in which she felt loved and protected. She tried desperately to make up for it when she finally had her own family. She sought this missing love from her husband and children, and clung to us so we almost felt suffocated. I felt that she was always breathing down my neck. And she was obsessively suspicious; she kept tabs on everyone I had contact with and even read my letters. I shut myself off from others more and more, and lived with miserable feelings deep inside myself; "Nobody understands me and I can't do anything right in the eyes of my mother – she accuses me of being lazy and doesn't realise that I can take initiatives of my own." Even today, I feel that she tried to bind us to the family psychologically – which, of course, had the effect of making me try all the harder to get away.

Erika saw no chance of getting support from her father. This was a mistake, but because his job had taken him away from the family for so many years she was somewhat estranged from him, and she had the impression that he always sided with their mother. Later in life, Erika's older sister said that he would probably have helped her, if she had not been so reserved and uncommunicative. Thanks to an intense exchange of letters, Erika and her sister, who was away studying in Berlin, managed to remain close during these years. The brothers, for their part, could stay out of their mother's "line of fire". The eldest was mostly away, and sensitive and withdrawn Ernst, three years Erika's senior, was largely left to go his own way, probably out of fear of hurting him. So Erika had to endure the pressure alone, and the first signs of the endogenous depression which was to recur throughout the greater part of her life gradually become noticeable.

However, there were also sources of happiness during her adolescence. Her growing love of music – singing, and playing a musical instrument – which was awakened and fostered by her musician sister, Trudi, brought her increasing joy. And most important of all were the Bible study and confirmation classes with Rev. Schulthess. The classes meant a great deal to her, and it was here that she met a dear friend and confidante, Julie. But Erika's mother – who was genuinely concerned about her daughter's inner development – was afraid that both Rev. Schulthess and Julie were having much too much influence over her, and that this was not good, and might well alienate her daughter from her. From the point of view of the bourgeois morality of the day, there were reasons for both of them to be considered objectionable – though this was not openly expressed. Julie was seen as an illegitimate child, because she had grown up in the care of her aunts, and was therefore seen as undesirable as a contact for Erika. And Rev. Schulthess was divorced – that was unimaginable for a man of the Church! Indeed, soon after Erika's confirmation, he gave up his profession.

Yet the biggest burden on Erika, and the rest of the family, was that her mother suffered for years from intestinal bleeding. A physical basis for the illness was never found. In Erika's experience, it was a means of exerting pressure and having power that came into action whenever her daughter became involved with anything outside the family. When she went out anyway, instead of staying at home and caring for her mother, she had to wrestle with feelings of guilt and resentment. Against this background, it becomes easier to understand the feelings of depression and anxiety about the future that Erika experienced at the end of the journey her class made at the end of their time in school.

Despite the difficulties of life at home, Erika is still thankful for the many intellectual and cultural ideas to which she was exposed there. Her mother's social engagement as president of a women's association to encourage abstinence from alcohol made a strong impression on her. Her father made his mark on the life of the family through his wide-ranging interests, particularly in politics and literature. The family often shared a special interest – for instance in a particular author. Erika remembers how this often showed up at Christmas. When they all opened their presents they often found that everybody had secretly decided to present the others with a book by the same author. One year it was Adalbert Stifter, and another year Jakob Burckhardt

III University Studies during World War II and starting in a profession

The challenge of choosing a career

In 1936, Erika had finished High School with the Cantonal *Matura*. Now she could take any course at the University except medicine or pharmacy, which both required Latin. What should she choose?

The apple doesn't fall far from the tree – natural sciences?

Looking back on her academic performance and preferences, Erika says she was especially good in subjects related to the natural sciences, maths and German, but was very bad at foreign languages. Yet she eventually went on to write books in English, she notes with a mischievous laugh. In those days, it was unusual for a girl to show talent almost exclusively in the natural sciences, which occasionally made her feel like an outsider. But her specific interests were underpinned by family tradition: her father was a chemist, her older brother Hans was a radio technician, and her younger brother Ernst would one day become a well-known ornithologist. She had already discovered her own deep love of flowers and plants as a young child in the vacation paradise of Troistorrents, Valais, and began collecting and naming them systematically with the "plant Bible", the authoritative Swiss Flora by Dr August Binz.

Awareness of social disparities and problems

Though she grew up in a sheltered middle-class environment, Erika's family had a great deal of sympathy for socialist ideas. Erika became familiar with the struggles of the socially disadvantaged at an early age thanks to her older sister Trudi's social engagement, and she gradually developed a keen sense of social disparities. In the primary school she noticed, for example, that one of the little girls always wore dresses made of the grey-striped "school cloth" subsidised by the city for children from impoverished families. She began for the first time to realise what social discrimination stemming from poverty could mean. She often used to tag along when Trudi was helping to organise recreational activities for working-class children in the industrial district of Basel, as a member of a group called "Ulme", which had been founded by members of the circle around Leonhard Ragaz, the pioneer of religious socialism.

Trudi used to bring some of the children back with her to Lenzgasse, where Erika played with them in the familiar surroundings of her family home. Such experiences helped to provide the basis for Erika's own social engagement later in life. During the years leading up to her confirmation, Erika became actively involved in youth work in the church. Among other things, she and her friend Julie took on the leadership of a group for socially disadvantaged youngsters from the St. Johann neighbourhood. Working on behalf of her parish church, she regularly visited an elderly woman living in heart-rending circumstances. Finally, she and a few school friends founded a group they called "POU", which stood for *Pfadfinderinnen ohne Uniform* (Girl Guides without Uniforms), dedicated to being kind and helpful not only when wearing a uniform – like the traditional Girl Scouts – but at all times. But today she admits, with a laugh, that she didn't always manage to live up to this ideal, especially at home – much to her parents' disapproval.

The search for religious guidance

Was it the absence of Christian socialisation at home that made Erika so receptive to the religious currents of her day, spurring her to seek out her own faith? Already as a small child she had enjoyed listening to the biblical stories read by her nanny Lydia Bitzer. Though Erika's father identified himself as agnostic, he wanted his children to receive church-based religious instruction, so they could eventually make their own well-informed decisions regarding matters of faith. There was one condition – the lessons shouldn't be taught from a religiously conservative point of view. So Erika attended classes in religious instruction with a decidedly liberal pastor, Rev. Ernst Schulthess. As a result, in her formative years she intensively pondered questions of Christian faith and was actively engaged in youth work through the liberal *Zwinglibund* (called after the Swiss reformer, Zwingli). She enjoyed reading religious literature, especially some rather pietistic biographies. Her interest was also captured by the high moral values espoused by the "Moral Rearmament" movement centred in Caux in Switzerland. But could she really live up to such values? Erika was always keenly aware of her limitations.

Exploring a completely different part of the religious spectrum, Erika came across Christian Socialism. Copies of the magazine founded by Leonhard Ragaz, *Neue Wege* (New Paths), had been lying around in the family home in Lenzgasse ever since Trudi had begun subscribing to it when Erika was a child. In the light of her intense religious interest, it is only natural that after leaving school Erika considered studying theology, with the idealistic goal of bringing together the rival religious currents of conservative orthodoxy and progressive liberalism.

A decision is made

Erika took her time to make the decision about what to do next. After she left school she spent a year in Zürich where she attended a housekeeping school, which gave her thoughts about her career a chance to ripen. Finally, it became clear to her. Choosing between training as a social worker, studying theology, and studying natural sciences, she opted for the third, specializing in botany. She wanted to become a teacher, and, with an almost missionary sense of purpose, to help children to understand the beauty of creation.

Studying during turbulent times

And so, in 1937 – two years before the outbreak of the Second World War – Erika began studying at the university in her home city, Basel. She combined botany and zoology as major subjects, and took geography and physics as minor subjects. The proportion of women studying natural sciences was small, except in medicine. Erika vividly remembers the crowded classroom during lectures by Professor Adolf Portmann, a man whose strong personality impressed everyone and who went beyond the borders of his discipline – zoology – to integrate artistic and ethical aspects into his teaching.

One of her minor subjects, physics under the stern Professor August Hagenbach, proved to be a bit of a challenge. Erika remembers:

> During laboratory sessions, the professor would walk around among the students, pick out one or the other of us, and pose question upon question. I think we were studying optics when it

was my turn. At first, everything went fine, but then he asked a question I couldn't answer. I stood, perplexed, in front of the blackboard filled with formulae. Then he lit himself a cigarette, which gave me a moment to think, and, as luck would have it, the answer occurred to me. Later on, my classmates told me they'd trembled at my predicament. I'd had no idea at the time that he always used to light himself a cigarette just before completely losing his patience and flying into a fit of rage.

After completing her basic courses, Erika chose to focus on plant physiology for her major. In her second year of studies, she already got a job in the Institute of Botany as an assistant to Professor Max Geiger-Huber. Her work included helping with practical classes for medical students, and assisting the Professor with experiments on plant growth hormones, which had just been discovered. One of their experiments involved the European Cornel *(Cornus mas)*. Branches were exposed to different concentrations of the synthetic growth hormone heteroauxin, and the number of blossoms on each branch was correlated with the concentration of hormone. This study eventually provided part of the basis for Erika's doctoral work with Professor Geiger. She sums up her time with him dryly and succinctly:

> He talked a lot, but I was fond of him – in fact very fond of him. He liked me too. But he was married. And by the end of my work for the doctorate under his supervision there was no love lost between us. My dissertation focused on the uptake of the growth hormone heteroauxin by cucumber seedlings. To determine the hormone concentration in a solution, you had to spend an hour stirring a mixture of reagents in a test tube placed in a freezing combination of ice and acetone. I personally came up with the idea of constructing a little machine which would automatically stir things and measure the temperature at the same time. I worked on the idea together with a technician at the Institute of Physics. It turned out to be an ingenious little gadget – and Geiger began passing it off as his own brilliant idea whenever visitors came! In actual fact, when I was developing the device with the technician, the professor had repeatedly said it wouldn't work. That's how things often went at the university.

Hints of love stories?

Erika, who has remained single to this day, catalogues the "crushes" she had on people in her student days with scientific precision – but she names no names, referring to them as "Numbers 1–4". When asked to elaborate, she answered laconically, "I'm not going to tell you everything!"

No. 1 took a geography practical class together with Erika under Professor Fritz Jäger. One day, the students were told to work in pairs, and she – the sole woman – was left waiting to be picked at the end:

> Then No. 1 chose me, and the others chuckled a bit – they sensed I had a crush on him. It never went very far between us. But we exchanged glances across our papers. A couple of times I dropped my pencil from excitement, and he had to retrieve it each time. He would also take lecture notes for me when I was sick. But things didn't go any further than that, probably because he was a strict Catholic and I was very Protestant in my views.

No. 2 was Professor Geiger, described earlier.

No. 3 was also a botanist. The Institute of Botany had one photometer, and anyone who wanted to use it had to make a written reservation on a little blackboard. Erika once added herself to the list, and found when she came to make her measurements that someone has written below her name: *"Erica arborea, the bäumige"*. (This was a rather botanical joke; a play on the similarity between the word *"Baum"* meaning "tree", and a colloquial Swiss German term *"bäumig"* that meant "super".) The comment was the work of No. 3, a specialist on fungi, and he and Erika became close friends

> But his mother once told me that if I wanted to marry him, I'd have to marry her as well. She couldn't let him out of her sight, since he had a heart defect. She would always make sure the door to his bedroom remained open, so she could hear how he was doing. That scared me off. And, indeed, he wound up dying young, later, after our relationship was over.

No. 4 was another fellow student who took notes for Erika when she missed lectures. Her mother appeared to be impressed by him, saying, "He's such a dear, and religiously just right." But Erika apparently hadn't noticed that he had his eye on her.

Completion of studies in geography – Africa on the horizon?

A bit abruptly, but discreetly, Erika tried to change the subject: "That about covers my studies."

At that time, students who were considering becoming teachers could take the first examinations for a teacher's qualification during their time in the university. Erika took the first of these, for the secondary school teaching certificate, in 1941. In the geography part, she was unexpectedly tested on Africa. Two years later, in 1943, Africa turned up again in her doctoral examination, which included knowledge of her subsidiary subjects like geography. This time she knew the answer to every question, except the prevailing temperature on top of Mount Kilimanjaro:

> I knew that Kilimanjaro reaches six thousand metres. The average sea-level temperature in the tropics is 27 °C, and with each additional one hundred metres of altitude the temperature decreases by one-half degree. But, under the pressure of the exam, I couldn't manage the calculation. The answer is about –3 °C

These were small events – but they perhaps foreshadowed Africa's later significance in Erika's life. At the time, she had no idea that she would spend a large part of her life in South Africa – the native land of the *Erica* plant family!

Not quite as planned: the start of professional life

Between her doctoral examination in 1943 and the advanced teacher's certificate examination in the spring of 1944, Erika had a chance to spend the winter months working at the meteorological observatory in Davos with Dr Walter Mörikofer. In Davos, skiing was an essential part of the work: the scientists had to make various measurements while going up on the Parsenn cogwheel mountain railway, and, once at the top, the way down was on skis. It was a wonderful and instructive time for Erika, and she got along so well with her boss that she later returned to Davos between jobs simply to help Mrs. Mörikofer in the household.

The date of the advanced teacher's certificate examination was drawing near. To teach at the High School level, Erika needed to pass this examination – but to become a fully qualified teacher, she would have had to spend a year in a teachers' training college after finishing her degree. To enter the college, students had to have a medical certificate from the school doctor. When Erika went to see him, the doctor asked, "Do you really want to become a teacher?" Then he plainly tried to dissuade her. With her fragile health, in particular her recurring gall bladder problems, she would scarcely have a chance of getting a job – even with the best of grades compared with other, less-qualified candidates – due to reservations about her being allowed to join the official pension scheme. At that time, there was an over-supply of teachers. Erika took the examination anyway and, returning home afterwards, announced with a big smile, *"They don't want me!"* Even today, when she talks about the event, she laughs triumphantly.

There's a story behind this. When she was at the university, the advanced students were required to teach at various schools while the teachers were away doing military service on the Swiss border. As a highly motivated biology-teacher-to-be, Erika was assigned a class of fourteen-year-old girls at the girls' High School in Basel. The girls were interested in anything but natural history, behaved rudely, and took advantage of Erika's insecurity. She realised then that she was much too shy to be a teacher. And now, she had been offered deliverance, just at the moment when she had to take the final examination! But what should she become, if not a teacher? Ideally, she would have liked to work at an agricultural research institute. She was good at team work, and she knew that she would be well suited to such a job. Nonetheless, in those days a woman with a normal university degree – and no training in one of the Federal Polytechnics – did not stand a chance of getting that kind of post

In the end, Erika went to work in animal physiology in the pharmaceutical firm Roche, in Basel. Roche had developed a calcium supplement with vitamin C. Erika had to feed it to rats and then analyse their urine and faeces to determine what had been absorbed and what excreted. Her team discovered that, in certain cases, the calcium phosphate produced by the

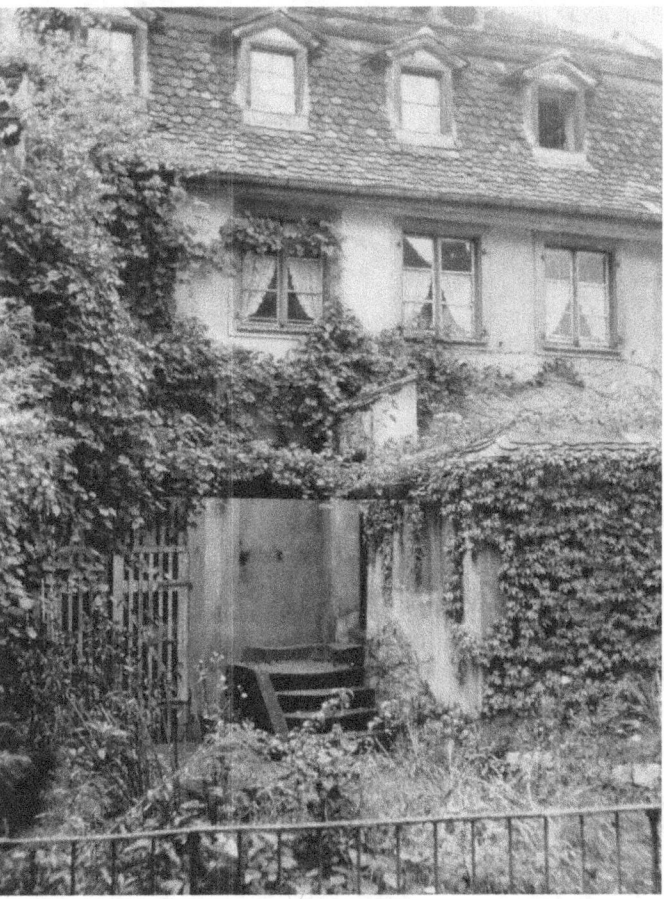

Spalenberg 20, where Erika lived with her sister, from the back, 1944

firm's competitor, Sandoz, was better, and they put this in the paper they prepared for publication in the renowned journal *Helvetica Chimica Acta*. However, before it was submitted for publication, the directors of Roche deleted everything from the text that might favour Sandoz. "And they called that science!" Erika is still indignant about it today.

Her boss at Roche was Dr Fromherz, who was German. He was well accepted by the team, even towards the end of the war. Once, during a daytime air raid on southern Germany which was so close to the border that the exploding bombs could be heard in Basel, he was heard to complain loudly about "those bastards!" meaning the Allies. Erika could understand his anger, considering that it was his country that was being destroyed.

Two unmarried daughters set up house on the Spalenberg

While she was working at Roche, Erika moved out of her parents' home in Lenzgasse to join her sister, who had recently moved into a flat in the Spalenberg, a steep little road leading into the old part of the city. For Erika, this was an important first step towards emancipation from her parents, enabling her to gain a little distance from her mother in particular. At that time, it was most unusual for unmarried daughters to move away from home. Trudi claimed that, as a music teacher, she needed to live closer to her students. And Erika had the good excuse that she could look after Trudi, who had serious health problems – and in addition, the journey from the Spalenberg to Roche was much shorter and easier. Erika's own health was not very good, even if the cause was psychogenic, as she believes in retrospect.

Their new freedom had its limits. On Sunday mornings, after the obligatory church service at the cathedral and a subsequent leisurely cup of coffee with friends in the Spalenberg, both daughters had to go to their parents' home in the Lenzgasse to cook lunch. It irked them greatly, and, in Erika's words, they sometimes said to one another:

> We could be married to the worst scoundrel in Honolulu, and that would be fine. But living together on the Spalenberg as two unmarried women is not considered suitable at all! They are always keeping an eye on us.

Trudi playing her violin, 1944

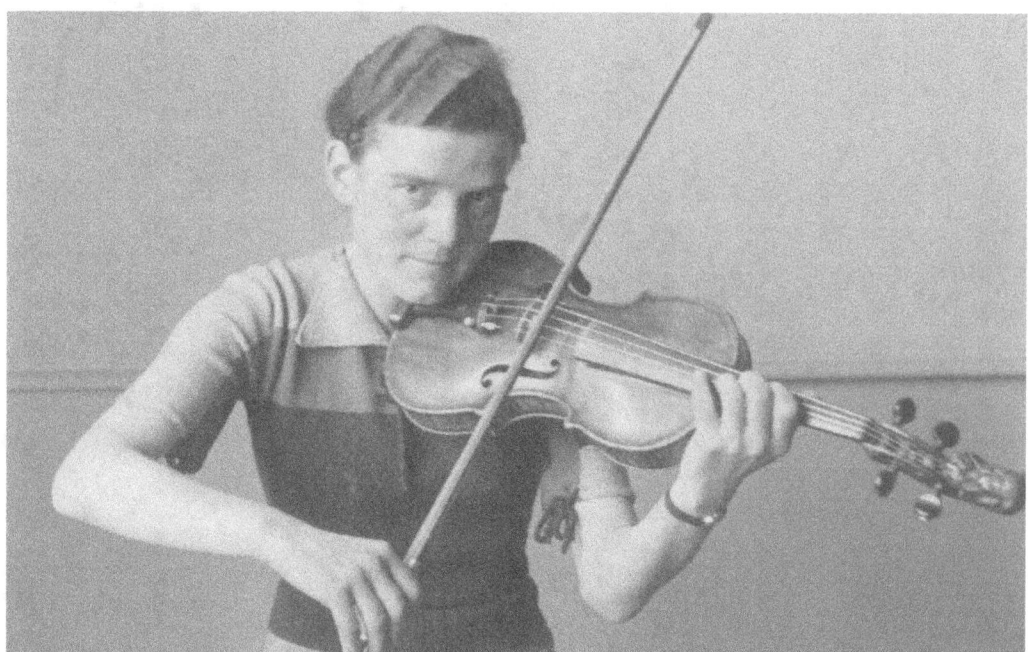

The time spent living with Trudi on the Spalenberg was a happy one. Through her sister, Erika immersed herself in the world of ancient music, particularly church music:

> Three prominent women musicians from the *Schola Cantorum Basiliensis* (a Conservatorium specializing in ancient music) – Ina Lohr, Lili Wieruzowski, and Trudi – collaborated on a big project. The aim was to make the wealth of hymns from the period of the Reformation, with their powerful texts and strong melodies, available for church services, small choirs and groups of singers, as a counterweight to the often sentimental hymns of Pietism. To that end, settings needed to be composed that people could sing and play. Ina took on the Lutheran hymns and Lili the Huguenot Psalms. Trudi was responsible for working on the hymns of Johannes Zwick, the leader of the reformation in Constanz. His hymns had fallen into oblivion, but Trudi discovered them in the library of the University of Basel. Wilhelm Vischer, a Basel theologian, rewrote the texts in a German that could be understood by modern congregations. I was intensely interested in the project, and it left its mark on me. To this day, since I know how briskly these hymns should be sung, I can't stand it when they are sung too slowly during church services.

Trudi maintained an open house in the Spalenberg. She took in a psychologically unstable music student for a period, and Jewish refugees from Germany were her most frequent guests. They were not only fed, but given a lot of attention and support in their difficult situation. Lifelong friendships were forged in that little flat. Trudi, energetic and clever, was brilliant in conversation and debate; Erika was not, but she was always present in the background. And, following Trudi's very untimely death in September 1945, Trudi's three closest friends became Erika's best friends. At one point, one of them remarked that before, she had simply seen Erika as an accessory to Trudi, but now she had come to see her as a person in her own right.

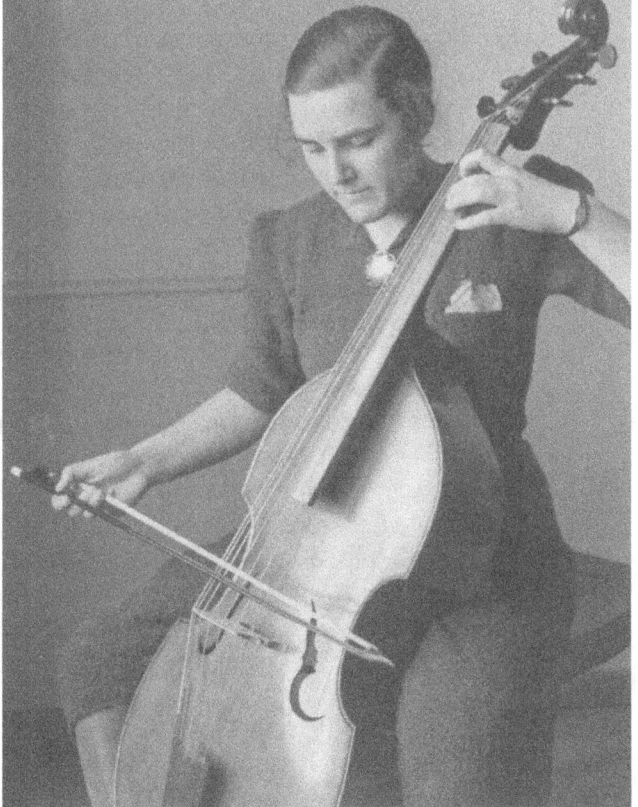

Erika with her bass viola da Gamba, 1944

Even after Trudi's death, Erika remained in the Spalenberg, much to the consternation of her parents – but it was absolutely crucial for Erika. Her brother Ernst began to come for lunch on a regular basis and the two of them taught themselves to cook. Erika remembers them turning the kitchen into a skating rink on one occasion, when they tried to cook spaghetti with one of the newly-introduced pressure cookers. One day, Ernst brought his future bride, Gaby, introducing her to Erika before anyone else in the family. It was only when she went to Sweden in 1948 that Erika gave up the Spalenberg, which was associated with so many good memories and important experiences.

Life during the Second World War

It is important to remember that these years of Erika's life – finishing high school and university studies, moving from the Lenzgasse to the Spalenberg, and working in Roche – took place against the backdrop of the Nazi era and the Second World War. What was her experience of this period?

> The period before the outbreak of war was very tense. At home, we followed the events with trepidation, especially England's initially hesitant stance towards Hitler. I can still picture Chamberlain's typical appearances before the media, with his umbrella in hand. When Hitler invaded Poland and I heard on the radio that war had broken out, I threw myself on the bed and began crying inconsolably into my pillow. Who knew what horrible events were to come? That moment is seared in my memory. I was caught between feelings of paralysis and powerlessness and the desire to do something useful. Then my PhD supervisor, Professor Max Geiger, told me about the volunteer air-raid protection troops, which were part of the Swiss defence forces. So I signed up, and was assigned to the Medical Corps as a medical orderly. Our boss was a likeable, somewhat shy doctor. I got along with her very well and she decided that, as an academic, I would make a good surgical assistant.
>
> The training to become a surgical assistant took two months at the cantonal hospital. That was my first contact with medical work; I had no idea then that I'd be performing operations myself one day! My first day working in the hospital was the first of August, which is a holiday in Switzerland, and it was pretty quiet. During the very first operation I was overcome with nausea at the sight of all the blood. That same evening the next emergency case arrived, and I had to jump in and assist. There was nobody else to help, so I couldn't allow myself to be sick again, and I got through it because I had to. I often thought back on this experience later on, when I was in the operating theatre as a medical student.
>
> Towards the end of the war, we were at last really able to use our medical skills. Numerous refugees from Alsace crossed the border into Basel, where they were given shelter in the big rooms of the Exhibition Centre (where Trade Fairs were held in peacetime). First, the new arrivals had to undergo delousing. DDT had just been invented. It was seen as a harmless insecticide and a real breakthrough for fighting pests, and we applied it generously – also to ourselves for our own protection. A first-aid station with beds was also installed at the exhibition centre. I remember there was a sweet old woman from Alsace, suffering from pneumonia, who was clutching a rosary and had a bottle of wine standing right beside her bed. She promised she'd invite us for an asparagus dinner after the war, to thank us for taking care of her – but we never heard from her again.

When war was declared in 1939, Erika was in the middle of her university course. She was not aware of any student groups that openly declared their political views, but she sensed little or no sympathy for the Nazis at the university – everyone in her immediate environment there appeared to oppose Hitler. But she had a geography teacher, Professor Jäger, who had been known for some time to be a National Socialist. Before the war this had not been seen as a serious problem, but when the war had begun, and he came into the lecture hall and hung up a map showing Switzerland as a part of Germany, charges were brought against him. Erika was asked to be a witness, but in the end she was not called to appear in court. Professor Jäger was forced to leave Switzerland in 1947.

Life in Basel was very much affected by the war. Food was rationed, and although Switzerland was neutral, there was a compulsory blackout to prevent pilots orienting themselves by the lights of cities. There must be no street lighting, and all windows must be covered with black curtains. All the parks and gardens were dug up for the cultivation of vegetables. Many people in this exposed corner between the borders of France and Germany were afraid of an invasion by the German army. A little rhyme that was current among German soldiers circulated among the air-raid protection troops: *"Die Schweiz, das kleine Stachelschwein, das nehmen wir auf dem Rückweg ein!"* ("Switzerland, that little porcupine – we'll take it on the way back home!")

The fear of an invasion was especially acute on one particular night, when it appeared that the German army might break through the Maginot Line. The whole area was on high alert. (It was later revealed that several Swiss National Socialists, members of the Fifth Column, had been arrested. They had been caught with explosives, prepared to blow up bridges in the border area.) The members of Erika's air-raid protection unit were instructed to sleep in their uniforms – complete with boots – with their helmets and gas-masks beside them. Though nothing happened, it was almost impossible to sleep. Suddenly, in the middle of the night, one of the women began to sing a traditional Swiss song in her sleep: *"Uf em Bärgli bin i gsässe..."* ("I sat upon the mountain top..."), and it relieved the tension.

Though Switzerland was officially neutral, there were Allied bombers operating close to the border, and from time to time they dropped bombs in Switzerland. These incidents were always said to be accidental, but it seems unlikely that the Allies' knowledge of geography was that imprecise! Perhaps they were targeting the German coal trains rolling through Basel on the way to Italy, carrying weapons hidden underneath the coal. (Officially, no one knew anything about them.) The bombing of Schaffhausen and Neuhausen by the Allies on April 1st 1944 also seems hardly likely to have been simply coincidental. There was a Neuhausen-based company, SIG, that delivered weapons to the German Reich. The family home in Lenzgasse was very close to the French border, and the missiles practically flew over the house. Erika's father anxiously watched the fire-bombs falling on Lörrach, the German town that is adjacent to Basel, and worried about his family's fate, should the Germans invade. His wife was half Jewish, so the children were one-quarter Jewish. If the Germans had invaded, they would have been victims of the Nazi race laws, and might have ended in a gas chamber. It was the first time that Erika really became aware of her Jewish background.

An eyewitness account of Christian resistance in Basel and Switzerland's official stance towards the Nazis

In the experience of Erika and her sister Trudi, the churches in Switzerland vehemently condemned the policies and the supporters of Nazism. Both Erika and Trudi were regular church-goers and, throughout the 1940s, attended the services of three Protestant pastors known for their firm stance against racism. They were Walter Lüthi in the Oekolampad church, Wilhelm Vischer in St. Jakob's church, and Eduard Thurneysen in the Cathedral. All three were actively engaged against Nazism, in word and deed, and were kept under surveillance because it was alleged that they were communists. As Erika learned only recently, Rev. Lüthi and the Basel Professor of Theology, Karl Barth, were blacklisted by the Swiss secret service, and some of their writings were banned by the censors. In Erika's opinion, a great fear of communism and socialism dominated Switzerland at this time, which could have been one reason why the official position of the Swiss Federal Council was becoming more and more Nazi-friendly and right-wing. Switzerland was also maintaining a very restrictive refugee policy towards Jews, which affected Erika's and Trudi's Jewish friends.

The two sisters supported the anti-Nazi and no-more-war movements and proudly wore the "no more war" emblem depicting a broken rifle. Towards the end of the war, Erika's status as a corporal in the air-raid protection unit required her to spring into action in the event of an air-raid warning. But in one instance she didn't hear it, and another time she simply went back to sleep thinking that the alarm was in Germany. As nothing happened, she was not missed and there were no consequences!

However, on another occasion bombs did fall in Basel. Erika was off duty, and had accompanied her sister to the Bethesda Hospital, where she was to receive a blood transfusion. She was waiting in her sister's room, when she suddenly heard planes approaching, and looked out of the window. It was March 4th, 1945 – a beautiful sunny day. She saw "matchsticks" falling through the air, and the ceiling light suddenly crashed to the floor. She found out later that bombs had been dropped near the main Swiss railway station.

A slightly tipsy celebration at the end of the war

On the day the war ended, May 8th 1945, Erika cycled directly to the Lenzgasse after work as usual, to spend the evening with her sister. Trudi had been living back at home in the care of their parents for several weeks, because she was seriously ill – she was suffering from kidney failure.

The sense of joy and relief at the end of the war was immense. Cycling home through the darkness to the Spalenberg, Erika was stopped by a policeman because the light on her bicycle was out. She told him that she had forgotten to turn it on out of sheer happiness at the end of the war, and the friendly policeman told her to ride on. Only afterwards, when she was safely out of sight, did she realise that the bicycle light was actually broken.

The next day, Erika and two colleagues from the laboratory went for lunch at a nearby restaurant as usual. To celebrate the end of the war they shared about half a litre of wine – not much, but enough to make Erika feel "a bit tipsy". It was a new experience for her, as she was completely unaccustomed to drinking wine. She remembers the incident vividly:

> After lunch, I went about my usual measurements with the precision scales, but I had the strange sensation that it was someone else, not me, who was standing there weighing things.

Friendships with Jewish refugees

For the entire period following Hitler's seizure of power in 1933, and during and after the war, Jewish refugees from Germany passed in and out of the Spalenberg and the family home in Lenzgasse. Through them, Erika learned at first hand what was happening in Germany and began to take an interest in politics. Time and again, she saw the discriminatory manner in which the Swiss authorities dealt with Jews, and was critical and ashamed.

Our contact with refugees began with Annie Loebenstein. When Trudi was studying at the Academy for Church and Folk Music in Berlin in 1933, she had a Jewish teacher of music theory called Miss Loebenstein, whom she greatly appreciated. Trudi's teacher eventually converted to Catholicism and entered a very strict convent, which only allowed her to send one letter home a year and to receive one letter. In one of these letters, she learned that her niece, Annie, had fled to Switzerland and found a job as an assistant at the Institute of Physical Chemistry in Basel. Miss Loebenstein asked her niece to contact Trudi, so Trudi found out that Annie was in Basel. The two made friends immediately, and from then on Annie ate all her meals with our family at our parent's home, and she became an integral part of our lives. Much later she married a Belgian whom she met in Switzerland, and went to live in Brussels.

Trudi's special protégée was Lili Wieruszowski, a highly gifted organist, and a committed Jewish Christian. She had a lot to endure for many years. She had become a well-respected organist in Germany – and then, in 1933, she was forbidden even to lay a finger on an organ! That same year she fled to Switzerland. Here she was not permitted to work for pay, and was not given a residence permit. Until 1949, she lived in fear of being expelled from the country. The authorities remained obstinate, despite the efforts many people made to help her. I got to know Lili through Trudi, and after Trudi's death she became my best friend. We shared joy and pain with one another and stayed in close contact – even during my years in Africa – up until her death in 1972.

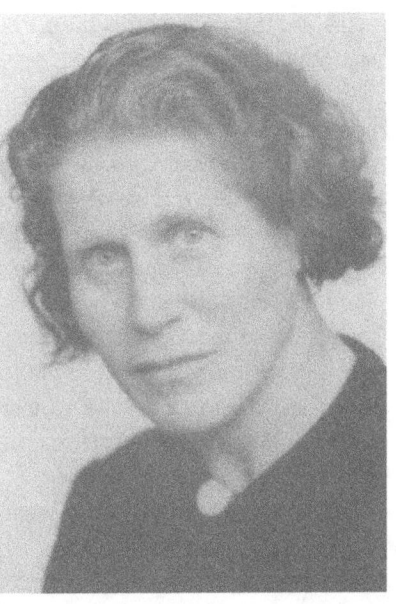

Lili Wieruszowski, who became Erika's best friend after Trudi's death, 1946

Through Lili, we also got in touch with a family of musicians called Strauss. They had managed with great difficulty to escape from German-occupied France and cross the "green border" (i.e. the part of the border that runs through the countryside) into Switzerland. The only thing they were able to save was Gertrud's violin. She crawled under the fence with the violin clasped to her stomach. Her two boys were taken in by a family in Basel, and my parents invited her and her husband to live with them on Lenzgasse. When the elder son wanted to learn to play the cello, but no one had money for an instrument, I lent him mine, since I was only playing the bass viola da gamba at the time. To this day, I'm proud that I enabled him to begin playing the cello. He became an excellent musician and eventually played as first cellist in the Basel Symphony Orchestra.

We had even more Jewish guests in Trudi's flat. One was Hugo Solms, whose parents had fled from Berlin to Holland. His father was a physician and had been head of the maternity clinic at the renowned Charité university hospital in Berlin. The two sons went to a boarding school in Switzerland and qualified for university studies. A wealthy Basel lady made it possible for Hugo Solms to study medicine. After Trudi's death he lived in a room in the Spalenberg for about a year. He completed the medical course, but because he was stateless, his examination results were considered invalid and he was not allowed to practice. Finally, after many years, he was able to become a Swiss citizen. In theory, in order to practice medicine even then he should have taken his examinations all over again – but he was let off, thanks to his fiancée's good relations with important people in the Swiss government.

And then there was a trip to Lisbon, which has a special story behind it:

During her time in Berlin, Trudi got to know a young man called Hermann Pflüge, whose wife was Jewish. They became close friends. The Pflüges emigrated from Germany to Lisbon in Portugal. Then Hermann wrote to Trudi saying that the family would have to move on and go to America, since things were becoming risky for Jews in Lisbon as well. So Trudi decided to use the school Easter holiday (she was giving violin and recorder lessons during the school term) to visit the Pflüges and their little daughter, who was her goddaughter. I was able to join her on the trip to Lisbon. It was April 1939. Most of our fellow-passengers on the ship from Le Havre to Lisbon were Jews who would be continuing on to America on the very same ship. On board, people also found out that Jews were being turned around and sent back from America. We heard terrible, tragic stories.

In Lisbon, there was only enough space for Trudi in the Pflüges' flat. I was given a room to sleep in at a Portuguese woman's home on a neighbouring street, and spent the days with Trudi and the Pflüges. One evening, we went to eat at a seaside restaurant. We had seafood, shellfish, and who knows what else, with *vinho verde*. In the middle of the night, I started to feel as sick as a dog. I began to review what I had eaten in my mind, and when I got to the mussels, I suddenly had to rush to the bathroom. It was full of large crickets, which scattered in every direction (crickets are sacred creatures in Portugal, and are offered for sale in the market). I relieved myself. My hostess was woken by the commotion and came to bring me a big pot of tea. She stayed with me while I drank the tea, mothering me with the utmost concern. When the teapot was nearly empty, she asked me something like *"mais?"* I didn't speak a word of Portuguese, but I assumed she was asking whether I felt better and I said "Yes". Then she brought me another full pot of tea! *"Mais"* meant "more"!

Aside from that experience, it was a lovely time. I would have been happy to stay longer in Portugal, even after Trudi had to return to Basel because school was starting. But a telegram arrived from our father, urging me to come home at once. He sensed that war was about to break out, and he didn't want me to get stuck in Portugal. He was right, of course. On the first of September 1939, Germany invaded Poland and the war broke out in all its brutal reality.

IV Preparing for Africa

First contact with the mission

After the end of the war, Erika continued to work in Roche in the animal laboratory, but she felt dissatisfied and began to look around for a new job. Then, simply by chance – or perhaps, as she believes today, it was God's guidance – an opportunity arose. A good friend of hers, who regularly came for tea in the Spalenberg, was Marie-Louise Martin. They had originally met at the Zwingli Association youth camps in Ticino, which Marie-Louise used to run. In the meantime, Marie-Louise had studied theology, and one day she announced as she sat at the tea-table: "This is the last time I'll be visiting – I'm joining the Swiss Mission in South Africa to work as a chaplain at a high school."

Marie-Louise mentioned in passing that Swiss teachers were always needed at this school. Erika began turning things over in her mind. Could it be God's will that she should volunteer for missionary service? Rev. Eduard Thurneysen, one of the pastors at the cathedral, encouraged her to do so. But if she was going to join a missionary society, it wouldn't be the Basel Mission. At the time, she felt it was too narrow and pietist. Another possibility was the Swiss Mission in South Africa, which had its headquarters in French-speaking Switzerland, in the *Département Missionaire des Églises protestantes* in Lausanne, but many groups of supporters in German-speaking Switzerland. The secretary of the Zürich office, Rev. Rippmann, was impressed with Erika's interest, and arranged for her to meet some missionaries who were at home on furlough, so that she could get a better idea of what missionary service would entail. Everything was off to a promising start – but then Erika's sister Trudi died in September 1945, followed by her father three months later. Erika did not want to leave her mother alone in such sad circumstances, so she went on working for Roche in Basel. In retrospect, she views this change to her plans in a positive light. Inwardly, she would not have been ready to leave and would have continued to suffer from health problems.

A circuitous route leads to a successful plunge

In 1948, a new opportunity appeared to open up thanks to Erika's friend, Annie Löbenstein; she could go to work for a Belgian professor of botany in Ghent, collaborating on a development project for Zaire. Erika handed in her notice at Roche, but learned shortly thereafter that the project's sponsor had backed out. However, by this time Erika definitely wanted to go abroad, preferably to Holland or Sweden, to work in a botanical institute. She was offered a job in Sweden, as a paid assistant in the botany department of the Swedish University of Agricultural Sciences, in Ultuna, near Uppsala. She says of this decision:

> I knew that I would enjoy the botanical work, and Sweden appealed to me – partly because of a book I had read as a child that really struck my fancy, called "A Teacher among the Lapps". So I accepted the job gladly. Nevertheless, I shall never forget the day when I had to bid farewell to Basel. As the train left, and my mother waved good-bye from the platform, I was overcome by a sense of certainty about one thing; I would never spend a long time in Switzerland again. Of course, my leaving wasn't easy for my mother, since my sister was no longer alive. For me, however, it was good to go. My frequent physical ailments disappeared, and in Sweden I regained my health.

Two happy years in Sweden

After a long journey by train and ferry, there she stood, on the platform of the railway station in Uppsala, waiting in vain for a Swiss student who was supposed to pick her up and take her to where she was going to live. Erika thought she would be impossible to miss with her cello tucked under her arm! But the student never came, and finally, with the help of a lot of gesturing, she managed to find her way to her landlady. She could scarcely speak a word of Swedish. During the first two weeks at the university, her colleagues spoke German with her – except for one professor who insisted on speaking to her in Swedish, but did so slowly and clearly. Looking back, she realised that this was very helpful, because she steadily became more and more comfortable with the Swedish language – she who thought she had no talent for languages! That gave her courage.

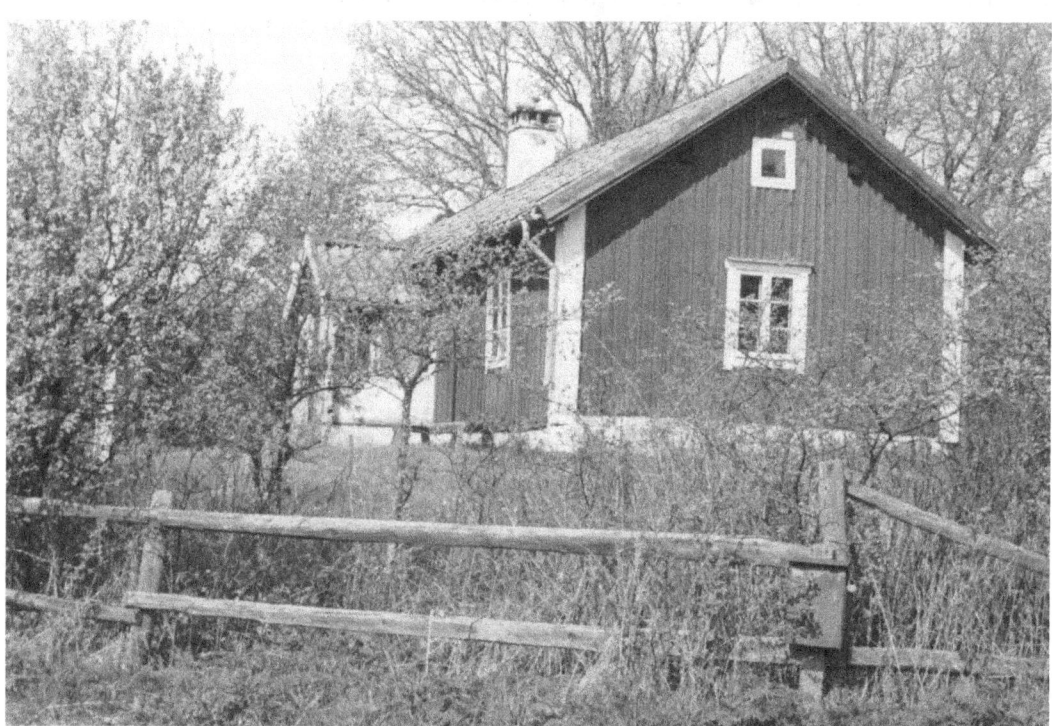

Erika's house in Penningby during her studies on young trees, Sweden 1949

Erika's research work at the beginning involved a study of the respiration of wheat roots. In the summer of her second year, she was given a new four-month assignment near Norrtälje, beside a picturesque bay with many little islands on its outskirts. There, she lived on the Professor's private estate, in his son's holiday cottage, and conducted research on capillary action in trees. To make measurements, she had to chop down and saw up small trees – something that would not have been allowed in Ultuna's state forest. In the course of this solitary work she enjoyed a wonderful friendship with the family of the pastor, Rev. Solén, in the village of Länna, twelve kilometres away. She very much liked the Soléns' daughter, who was about her age, but she was especially fond of their grandmother – the first grandmother she had ever known!

She soon began to spend every summer weekend in Länna, and was even invited to celebrate Christmas with the family. It was a very traditional affair, featuring red Yuletide ribbons, white dwarves, lots of candlelight, flaming torches in the snow, songs, and music from a harmonium waking everybody up for a church service at 6 a.m. – altogether, quite an experience. And above all, the traditional meals! On Christmas Eve there was a feast with a huge ham in broth, accompanied by Swedish gingerbread, beetroot salad, and for dessert, of course, rice pudding. A peeled almond was hidden in the pudding, and tradition had it that whoever found it would marry in the coming year.

Telling the story, Erika smiled at the memory:

> That year, somebody had dropped two almonds in by mistake – and they both turned up in my bowl. They must have neutralised each other; nothing came of it!

On Christmas morning, everyone in the house woke to the sound of the harmonium, and carrying torches they made their way through the deep snow to the festive service. Lunch consisted only of dried fish preserved with potash, which no one much liked – but everyone had to partake of it, for it was supposed to be good for the stomach. It was the traditional Christmas Day lunch everywhere in Sweden. To this day, Erika winces at the thought of it, but her eyes still light up at memory of those happy days.

After two years, it was time for Erika to leave Sweden. She did not do this by the most direct route; instead, she first went North on a long farewell trip through Sweden with a former schoolmate from Switzerland. They took a direct train to the north, to Lappland, where they had booked a place to stay at a bungalow-hotel in Abisko, the northernmost point along the train route from Kiruna to Narvik. From Kiruna onwards there were no roads, only footpaths, several lakes with boat connections, and a railroad. The regional doctor had a car outfitted with railway wheels, and drove along the railway lines. In the course of some very adventurous but well-organised hikes and ship crossings, the two young women resolved to visit a group of Lapps. A boatman invited them into his cottage – and while they were there, they suddenly realised that they'd missed the last passenger train to Abisko. "No problem," said their host, "all you have to do is hitch a ride with the next train carrying iron ore from the mines – they run every half hour – and ask to be let out at your hotel." And it actually worked! The friendly train driver even offered them tea and let them blow the train whistle before each tunnel. The goods train even made an extra stop right in front of the hotel to let them out, which caused a good deal of surprise in the hotel.

Their travels included a long journey on foot from one tourist hut to the next. In Sweden, it is a matter of course that each walker leaves the appropriate payment in a cash box in each hut. The snow was piled high in the area, and on a snow-covered field the two friends saw an animal walking back and forth.

Erika tells the story:

> My friend suddenly asked, "Didn't you say there are wolves in Lappland?" "Yes", I answered. We had a small pocket-knife with us and decided that a lone wolf surely wouldn't do us any harm – so on we marched. As we got closer, we saw that it was a young reindeer that didn't have its horns yet. We then followed the path further, from cairn to cairn; my friend in front, and me behind her. I was looking around every corner to make sure there were no bears. My colleagues had said there were bears in the area, and a bear would have certainly been worse than a wolf. But my friend simply marched on, and I said nothing. Half a year later, when we looked at the photos of our trip, my friend exclaimed, "Do you remember that day? I was terrified that we might come across a bear, but you weren't afraid at all!" Ha, ha! We had walked for a whole day, one behind the other, and each thinking the other was ever so brave!

The two years in Sweden were a good time to look back on. And Erika said later that without her experience there, she would not have been ready for Africa. In Sweden, she encountered for the first time the kind of hospitality that would be very important in her life in South Africa. In both countries, distances are vast, and when someone knocks on your door, it's only natural to invite them in and offer them a place to stay.

A decision, and a second contact with the mission

Perhaps the most important result of Erika's time in Sweden was that it was there that she experienced the final impulse to commit herself to becoming a missionary. A number of events encouraged Erika to make this decision about her future. In the first place there were pleasant encounters and illuminating discussions with Dr Ysander, a Swedish missionary doctor who had been in India. And one day, at the manse in Länna, she found Mrs. Solén packing boxes for her son who was about to depart for Belingwe in Zimbabwe, near the border with South Africa, as an agricultural missionary for the Church of Sweden. Erika thought to herself: "I could apply to the Swiss Mission in South Africa once more". Her health had improved in Sweden, and she was feeling completely fit.

So, when she got back to Switzerland she contacted the mission. However, when she applied for the second time, Rev. Rippmann was no longer interested. By the time she would be ready to travel abroad, she would be over the age of thirty-five, and no one was accepted once they reached that age. His argument was meant to console Erika's mother, who was afraid of losing a second daughter. But Erika's old friend Marie-Louise Martin, who was still working as a school chaplain in South Africa, would not let her give up: "Just apply directly to Rev. Badertscher in Lausanne!" The *Département Missionnaire* in Lausanne was the original and operational headquarters of the Swiss Mission in South Africa, and was responsible for appointments. Erika took her friend's advice – and then things began to happen very fast. A laboratory technician was urgently needed at the missionary hospital in Elim. Erika was essentially a biologist, of course, but the job should be no problem for a scientist with experience in animal physiology, which she had.

To prepare for the work, she completed six months of laboratory training in Basel in the university psychiatric hospital and in the medical polyclinic, as well as learning about X-ray technology at the hospital in nearby Riehen, and doing a general course on tropical countries in the Swiss Tropical Institute. She emerged professionally well prepared, and she had also read a lot about Africa. However, she did not have a chance to take a course to prepare her specifically for her future missionary service – there was simply no time. In those days there were no preparatory courses in Switzerland for volunteers bound for the Mission in South Africa. Such courses were introduced later, and before that, many future mission workers attended courses in Selly Oak, England. Erika recalls her formal acceptance by the Mission Council in Lausanne, just prior to her departure, as a particularly funny episode:

> We were assembled in a chapel, with chairs arranged in a circle. The members of the Council were seated all around me and I had to answer their questions. I was never particularly pious – for example, I'd never been a Sunday-school teacher. I had to leave the room while they discussed whether they wanted me or not. I was called again and they informed me that everything was in order and that I had been appointed. There followed a long, long period of prayer, during which I felt the urge to cough. I struggled to hold it back until the tears rolled down my cheeks, and afterwards, they congratulated me: *"Ah, c'est un moment très émouvant!"* (Ah, it's a very emotional moment!) Yet it was only the tickle in my throat that "moved me to tears."

What was it that finally motivated Erika's decision for missionary service? It was a long process of maturing, and included detours and obstacles which, with hindsight, she now regards as important and necessary. Time and again, she asked herself if God wanted her to go there. On one occasion Hugo Solms, one of the family's Jewish protégés during the war, tried to discourage her from going by arguing that now, after the Second World War and in the wake of a growing "black consciousness", various liberation movements were emerging and, as a European, she would not be welcome in South Africa. But even this did not weaken her conviction: "This is my path". She did not see it as her calling – or as a vocation, in the language of piety. That was a term that she and her friend Irène Bourcart, who also worked for the Swiss Mission in South Africa, regularly scoffed at. It was not a matter of personal ambition, either. It was simply her path.

Final preparations and departure

Along with her contract, Erika received a long list from the *Département Missionnaire* in Lausanne of things she must purchase for her first tour of duty. "A real dowry, just as if it was a wedding", she says now. She could obtain pyjamas, sheets, and such things from voluntary associations of mission supporters in French-speaking Switzerland, whose members used to knit and sew useful items for departing missionaries. And, in view of the warm climate, Erika's mother sewed her some very pretty white laboratory overalls that could also be worn as light dresses. All her gear was packed into the solid boxes which missionaries – whose salaries were very modest – often put to good use as furniture in their country of service. Later, Erika would also equip her little home in Elim with packing-case furniture.

Shortly before Erika's departure there was a special service in St. Leonhard's Church in Basel, where Erika was given a blessing for her work with the mission. It is her wish that one day the circle of her life will be closed by a funeral service in the same church. One of the people she invited to the farewell service was a close student friend, who had shared Erika's time of preparation for the mission. But she was a devout Catholic, and had just been admitted into the Brother Klaus congregation in Stans, so – as was common in those days – she had to obtain permission from the church authorities before she could enter a reformed church, and it was only at the last minute that she was finally given permission to participate in the ceremony.

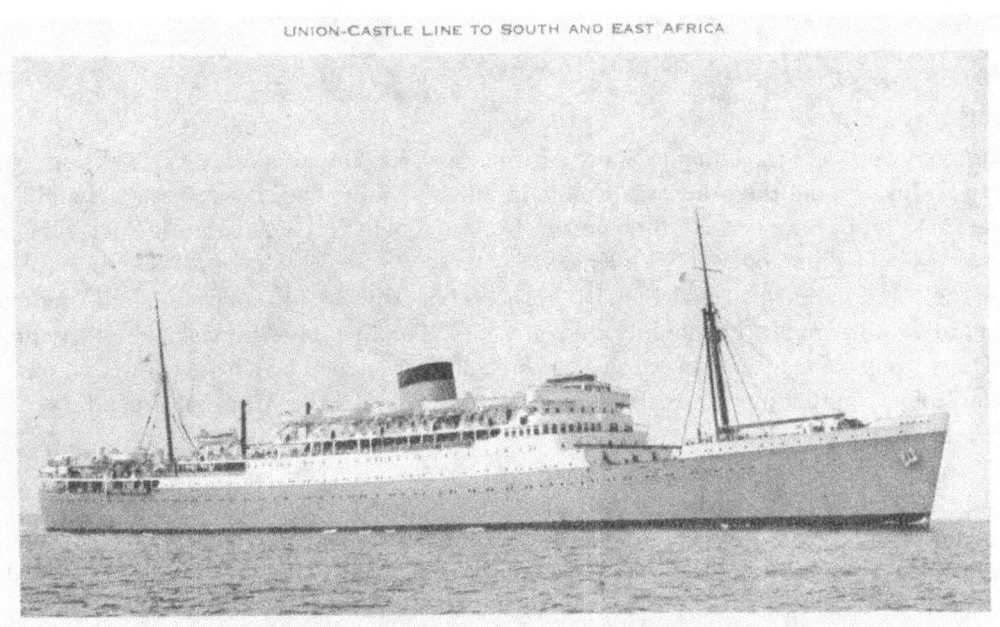

The "Warwick Castle", Union Castle Line, 1952

For Erika, the day remains a very happy memory:

> Rev. Eduard Thurneysen preached on the text I had requested, the Psalm of Christ in the Epistle to the Philippians, chapter 2, verses 5–11. I was blessed by Rev. Badertscher from the *Département Missionnaire*. I felt that this blessing would give me the strength to face whatever lay ahead in the foreign land. Even then, I knew that the hospital in Elim was not going to be a place of easy-going fellowship.

In mid-April 1952, Erika embarked from the British port of Grays in Essex. The *Warwick Castle* was not one of the big, fast ocean liners; she was an older, so-called "intermediate" ship belonging to the Union Castle Line, and it was her final voyage that took Erika to Cape Town in three weeks. Missionaries would continue to be transported by sea up to the late 1960s, since it was cheaper than flying. On board with Erika were four fellow-missionaries, a young married couple, Hans-Jakob and Nelly Walder, who were going to Mozambique, and two sin-

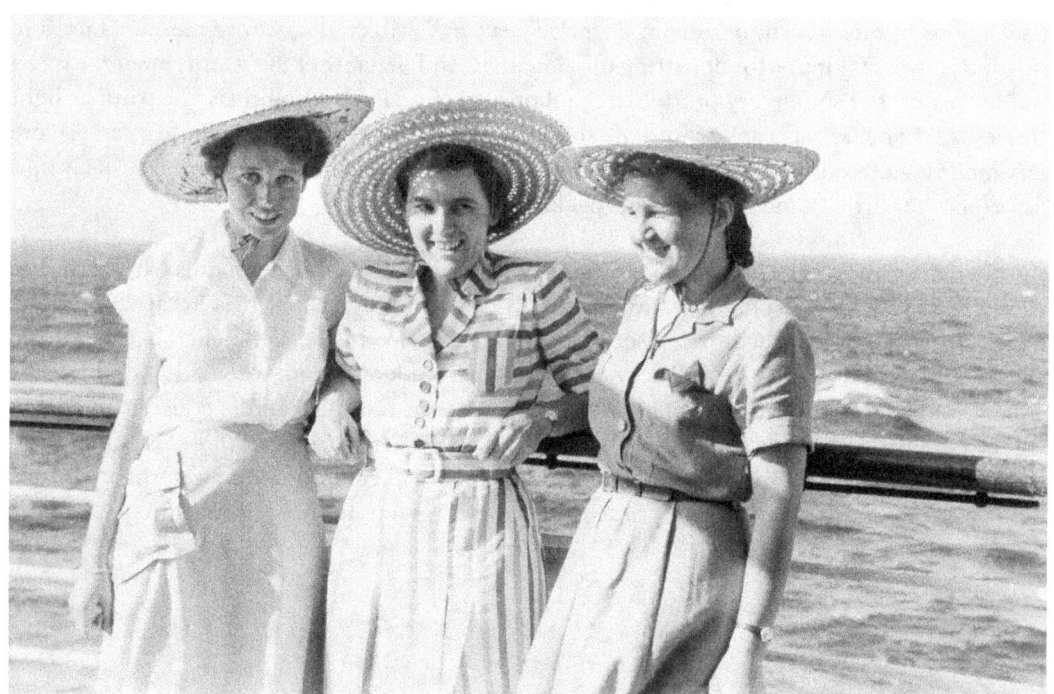

On the ship "Warwick Castle" on the way from England to South-Africa; from left: Nelly Walder, Erika, Ruth Keller

gle women who were travelling to South Africa like Erika. One was Ruth Keller, a nurse going to Shiluvane, and the other was Emma Fröhlich, who was over sixty years old and had come back from a long period of missionary work in China. She was venturing out to begin all over again in Elim, together with Erika.

After the hectic period of preparation, the leisurely boat trip was like a vacation for Erika, and she recalls with a smile, "I could idly enjoy myself". The five missionaries had fun together. And they made some interesting excursions on land that opened up a new world for them. It was in Lobito, on the Angolan coast, that they first set foot on the African mainland:

> A taxi brought us from Lobito to a small village in the interior. When we passed by a sugarcane plantation, our driver stopped, cut some sugarcane, and gave it to us in little pieces which we sucked on for the rest of the drive. Once in the village, the taxi driver brought us to a Catholic missionary school and explained to the teacher who we were. A throng of children quickly gathered around us and sang a song with their eyes beaming. This was Africa, up close and personal!

On a postcard from Lobito dated June 3rd 1952, Erika wrote to a friend, "Today I shook hands with a black person for the very first time." To this day, this handshake with an African teacher means as much to her as the blessing ceremony in Basel.

After three weeks, the *Warwick Castle* arrived at the port of Cape Town. The Walders were continuing with the ship to Mozambique, but the other three missionaries spent a few days in Cape Town before taking a train to Johannesburg, where they were met by another missionary, Rev. Büchler, with whom they stayed for a short time. Here they made some final purchases, particularly bedding and mattresses, and then it was time to continue on by train to Pietersburg (now Polokwane), where they were collected in small lorries and brought to their destinations, Shiluvane and Elim.

Perched among suitcases and mattresses at the back of the lorry from Elim Hospital, Emma Fröhlich and Erika rode along the unpaved road leading to Louis Trichardt in a cloud of dust. The landscape was very different from what Erika had imagined – a dried-out, flat and featureless grey-brown plateau, with nothing special about it. It was winter, of course. But then, shortly before Louis Trichardt, they took a turning to the right and Erika saw the beautiful landscape around Elim, reminiscent of the Swiss Jura. She felt very relieved to discover that she would be living in such a lovely region. The final stretch of the journey led up a hill to the hospital grounds. The hospital complex, made up of scattered single-story bungalow-style buildings, looked like a village to Erika. At the top of the hill stood the oldest building, the hospital for Europeans, and it was here that the journey came to an end.

It was June 13th 1952, exactly one day before Erika's thirty-fifth birthday. She couldn't resist having the satisfaction of sending a card to Rev. Rippmann in Zürich immediately, informing him that she had begun her missionary work in Elim before she reached the age-limit of 35.

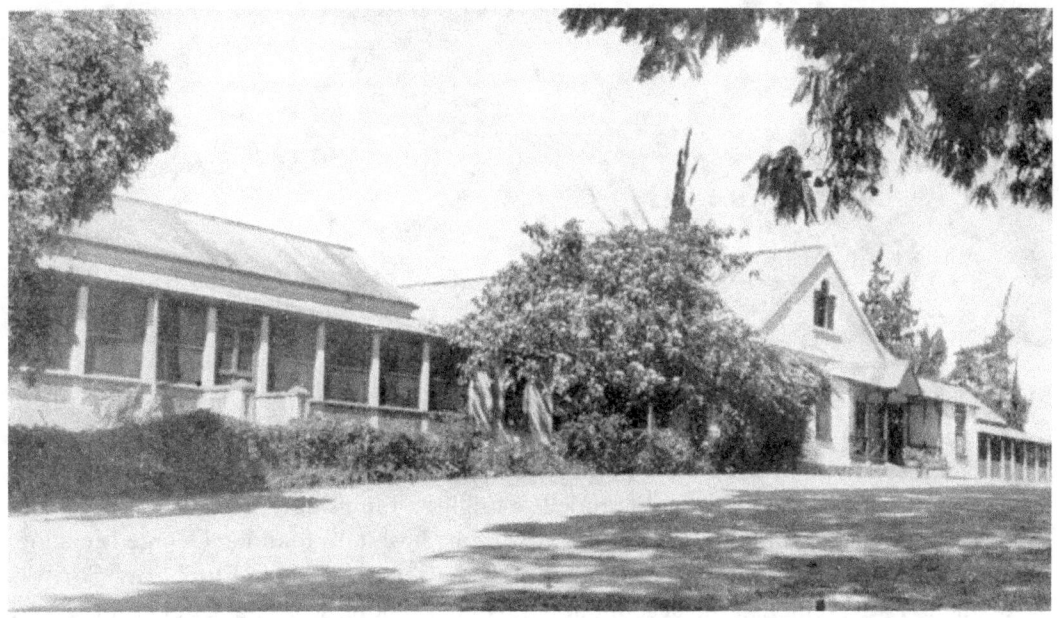

Elim Hospital, 1973. European Hospital and Administration Block and Indian Section

V The Path to Ophthalmology

Settling down in Elim

Upon her arrival in the hospital, Erika was greeted and taken to her room by Marie Näf, a small, sturdy woman with a warm presence. She was the hospital's head of domestic services. She immediately gave Erika her first instructions on dealing with Africans: "Make sure you never leave scissors lying around; they're a favourite item to pinch!" Erika was a little surprised at this attitude – but later, she learned to appreciate Marie Näf a great deal. She was responsible for the household and the kitchen, and she was very dedicated to the Africans who worked for her. She even founded a night school where she taught them basic reading and writing skills. She herself had only ever received a rudimentary education back in Switzerland; nevertheless, she was a remarkably knowledgeable and open person with diverse interests, and was someone with whom Erika could discuss theological questions or sophisticated books – a rare pleasure in Elim.

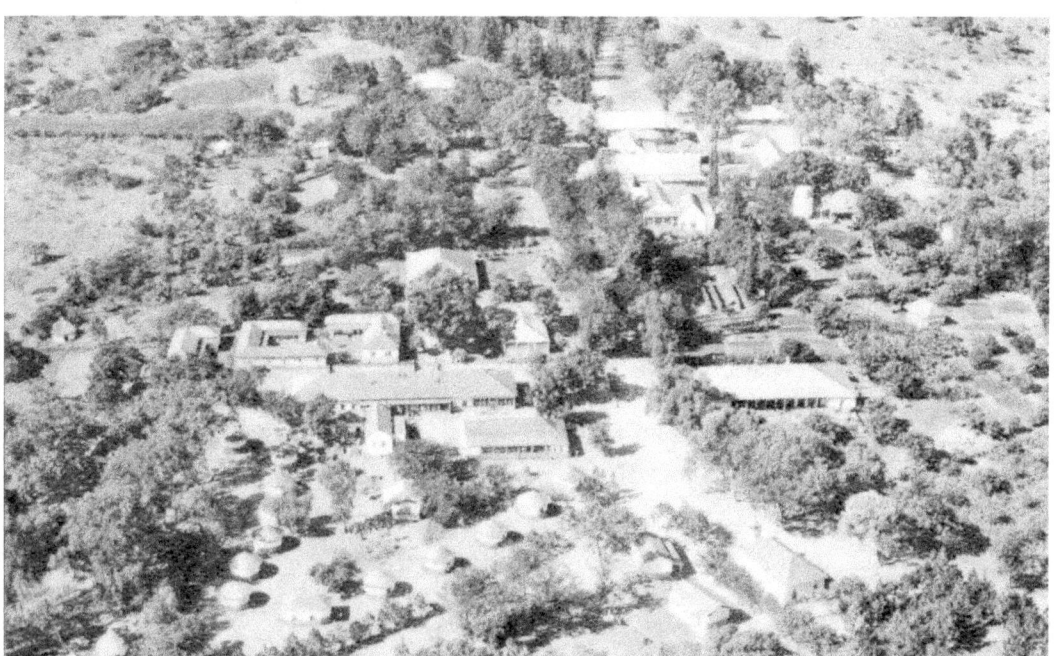

Aerial view of Elim Hospital (west – east), 1969

Already on her second day, her birthday, Erika had to begin work in the laboratory. Early in the morning, Madame Berthe Girardin burst in and placed a small vase of roses on the table, telling her that she could keep them during the day – but for the night shift she'd like them back, please! It was a kind gesture, intended to brighten things up, for life in Elim was not exactly easy. Madame Girardin was the daughter of the hospital's founder, George Liengme. Despite her advancing age, she still did night duty in the hospital for Europeans. She was nicknamed "La Reveilleuse" on account of her habit of waking sleeping patients at the start of her night shift, only to ask them if they would like a sleeping pill ...

On her first day, Erika was approached by Sister Fogelweid – nicknamed "Vögel" ("bird" in German) – who was in charge of the medical ward. She was known for her strict regime, and she informed Erika that she would be expected to deliver the test results from twenty or more urine samples every day by 10 a.m. As time went on, Erika found out that she was very competent and loyal, and was respected – even loved – by her African nursing students. Erika also immediately made the acquaintance of Sister Marquis, "La Marquise" – the woman with the sharpest tongue. The two got along quite well. It was often "La Marquise" who helped Erika late at night in the lab. She even used to bring along her gramophone and delightful albums of classical music.

Gradually, after the initial fleeting impressions, the faces that Erika encountered began to acquire deeper, and unexpected, contours. People's names were something she had to learn to get right. A particular complication was that whereas in German-speaking Switzerland nurses were called "Nurse so-and-so", using their first name, in Elim Hospital, as in French-speaking Switzerland, they were addressed as "Mademoiselle" followed by their last name. However, their last names were typically modified into a more endearing variant, like "Vögel", or "Marquise", or "Cavinette" for Mademoiselle Cavin.

The exchanges between the nurses were often sharp-tongued and brusque, but Erika quickly recognised that the cold façades masked good hearts, and that people's gruff exteriors were simply a means of coping with tough everyday reality. Nevertheless, the community could be difficult for the more sensitive. In her first weeks on the job, Erika quickly found herself lending a sympathetic ear to those who were having a rough time, providing a buffer between extremes, and she felt that this could become an important role for her in the future.

The origins of Elim

Before going any further, it would be good to take a brief look at the history of the Elim community. Dr Georges Liengme, a physician from Neuchâtel in Switzerland, founded the hospital in 1899. He had given up his post as a missionary doctor in Mozambique, and the Swiss Mission in South Africa sent him to work in the Transvaal Province. He made the difficult journey by ox wagon from Pietersburg to Elim, where a mission station had been established in 1896. There was a church, and a house for the pastor, and – most importantly – an excellent water supply. Water came from a well on higher ground, near the Lemana mission station.

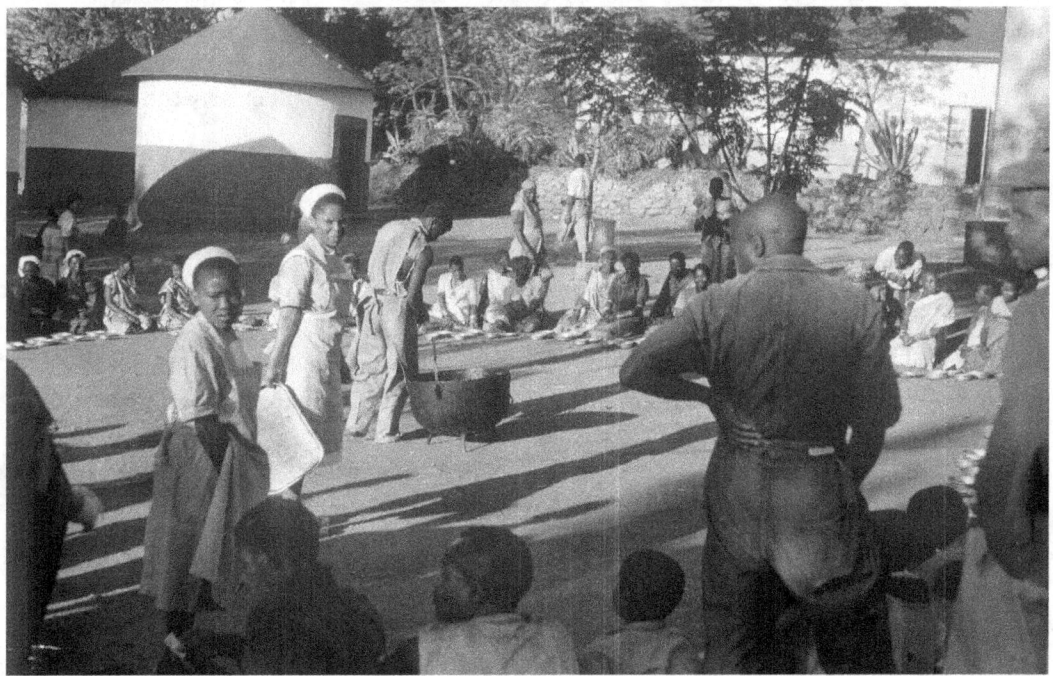

Lunch for the "village patients", those not needing a bed in the wards, but living in the rondavel in the hospital grounds, 1953

A missionary called Alexis Thomas built a water-mill, where the local people could bring their maize to be ground. The mill was still operated by the Thomas family when Erika was in Elim. Later, a small hydroelectric power plant was built in the same place, which provided electricity for the whole mission station.

The excellent water supply provided a good basis for Dr Liengme to establish a first little clinic there for the Africans. After a few years, the president of the Boer Republic, Paul Kruger, asked him to build a hospital for Europeans, because malaria had become widespread and was also prevalent on Europeans' farms in the region. This European Hospital – with around ten rooms for patients, a small operating theatre, a consulting room and the necessary ancillary rooms – exists to this day, and was one of the first buildings in the area to become a protected national monument. It sits at the very top of the hill, while the much more extensive hospital for Africans is housed in a number of pavilions further down the hill. There was also a small annex for Indian patients, which had been added to the European hospital by the members of the Indian community in Louis Trichardt. European patients were accommodated in the European hospital. For laboratory tests and X-rays they had to be preferentially treated. Looking back, Erika comments:

> For the medical staff, it was always hard to accept that the Medical Superintendent devoted far more time to the handful of European patients than to the larger "African hospital". It was true that in a roundabout way, the "European hospital" helped to finance the African hospital. Nevertheless, working in the European hospital remained a bone of contention among the European nurses and doctors.

A newcomer to a European settlement area

Erika arrived in Elim half a century after its founding, and she observed her new surroundings with a sharp eye. In truth, she was a little disappointed. In contrast to the way she'd imagined it, Elim was not located in the middle of the African bush; instead, it directly bordered the area settled by Europeans. The former thornbush savannah had initially been cleared by Europeans; Afrikaner and British settlers, and the descendants of Swiss missionaries. They mainly raised livestock, but as well as extensive pastures there were a few maize and peanut plantations. Among the descendants of the first missionaries were the members of the extended Thomas family, the farmers who had built the mill. They were still closely connected with the mission station.

By the time Erika arrived in Elim, the hospital had been subsidised by the state for several years. Racial segregation had already been imposed under colonial rule, and was systematised by law after 1948. Erika experienced every day the way that segregation affected the work of the hospital.

Erika's room was located in an annex of the European hospital in which a handful of European nurses were housed, though the majority of them lived in the hospital's original nurses' home – which was known as *Chantepleure* (French for "sing and cry"). It was so named because the Swiss residents would sometimes weep with homesickness, only to sing happily when their joy returned. The African nurses lived and ate in their own separate building, while the dining room for the European nursing staff was in the European hospital.

At these mealtimes, Erika noticed for the first time that the German Swiss and the French Swiss staff members – divided about equally in number – did not always get on with each other. Even before she left for Elim, she'd been told that it was a *"nid de guêpes"* – a wasp's nest. Sometimes, the members of the two groups would end up by chance sitting at separate tables, so the German speakers could happily speak their own language – Swiss German. But some of their French-speaking Swiss colleagues would criticise them for speaking a language they couldn't understand. Erika saw some justification for their resentment. The German-speaking Swiss only needed one language, French, to communicate with the others, and they had learned it in school. But the various dialects of Swiss-German are very different from the High German that the French-speakers had learned in school, and also from each other – and in addition, during Hitler's reign, it had been difficult for the French Swiss to use German at all, because if they spoke the High German they'd learned at school they were quickly decried as "Nazis".

Erika also remarked that:

> It was only in Africa that I really began to understand the Swiss peculiarity known as the *Röstigraben* – the linguistic and cultural gulf between the French- and German-speaking Swiss. (The *Röstigraben* is called after a fried-potato dish that is a particular favourite in German-speaking but not French-speaking Switzerland.) And I also had to travel to Africa to learn to play the Swiss card game "Jass", as well as how to cook fondue, which we sometimes ate on special occasions. .

From the start, Erika was assimilated into Elim's church life. It began with learning where she was supposed to sit. The pulpit was located at the front on a small platform, and there were benches on either side of it for the Europeans, while the Africans sat separately further down in the nave. Erika felt somewhat odd and conspicuous in her elevated seat, but accepted it as part of the situation and gradually got used to the fact that South Africa's racial fissures extended through church life as well.

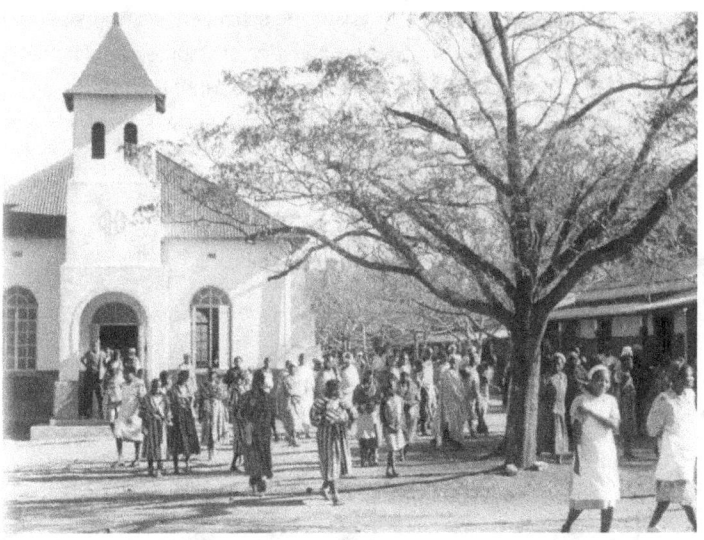

Sunday at the hospital. Patients and nurses after the service, 1953

For the Europeans, the daily hospital routine began at 6:30 a.m. with a morning prayer before breakfast in a small room of the main building. Morning Prayer for the Africans was at 7:00 a.m. in the chapel. The Europeans also met every Tuesday for an evening of prayer. Someone presented a meditation on a Biblical theme, and the evening closed with an open prayer session. The prayer meetings were held in different places in turn; at the hospital, at the mission station, at the nearby mission school, Lemana, or on a farm belonging to one of the descendants of Swiss missionaries living close to Elim. On occasion, Erika also had to lead such an evening. She remembers it as rather amusing:

> Whenever I interpreted a text according to my convictions, in the manner of the Swiss theologian Karl Barth, it was something of a contrast to the pietist Christianity of most of the others present. They used to use the open prayer period to submit to the Lord everything they had against my interpretation.

At Elim Hospital, the European Sisters would take turns leading a Bible Study evening once a week for the African nursing-school students. Erika greatly enjoyed this task and sensed that the young African women appreciated her. Perhaps it was partly because she sang with them so often and with such enjoyment?

For their part, the African students were responsible for the Sunday school for the hospital's littlest patients. Here, with African flair, the children were encouraged to act the stories, and plays were rehearsed to be performed at church festivals like Christmas. The church services for hospital patients were led by African evangelists or European missionaries. Members of the church women's organisation, *Vamanana* (which means "the mothers"), often paid bedside visits to patients.

Many of these activities were dominated by a pietistic style of Christianity, and Erika sorely missed a more lively spiritual debate and discussion of matters of faith. There was no place for questions or doubt, or for the kind of discussion she had been accustomed to. In a letter she wrote in December 1952 she thanked a friend for giving her the book "Letters and Papers from Prison" by Bonhoeffer. "It is like a piece of wholemeal bread in Elim's pietistic pudding," she wrote.

> Maintaining close contact with old and new friends at the nearby Lemana mission High School became all the more important for Erika. The school chaplain was her old friend, Marie-Louise Martin – the person who first gave her the idea of volunteering for missionary service. A good friend of Erika's from school, Irène Bourcart, also taught there, and through her she made more friends; Els Ziegler, who taught science at Lemana, and Louise Ulrich, who was in charge of the

View from Lemana, looking towards Elim down the valley, 1981

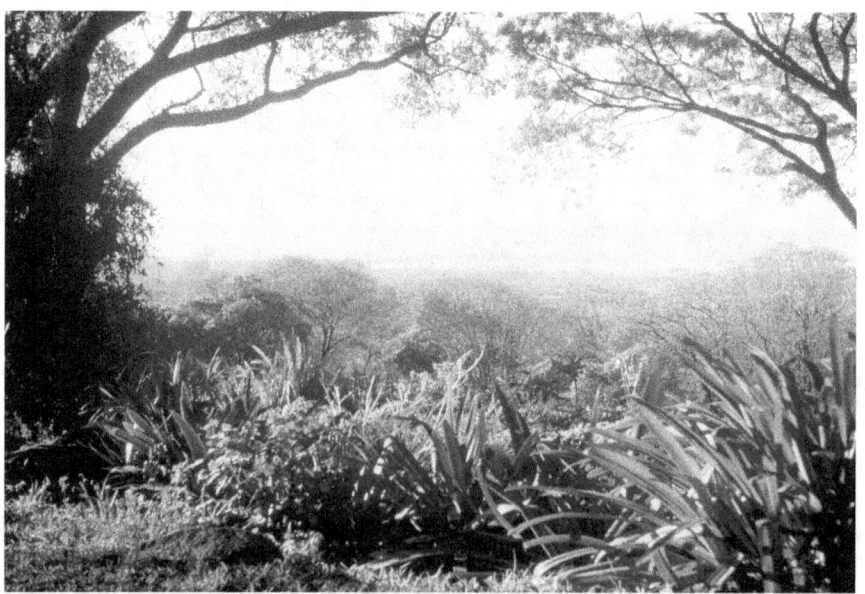

hostel for girls. The name Lemana, incidentally, was chosen by French-speaking Swiss missionaries who were remembering Lac Léman (known internationally as Lake Geneva). In fact, the landscape does bear a certain resemblance to the Swiss Jura, and at night, when the lights of Louis Trichardt could be seen in the distance, it was possible for Erika to imagine looking across Lake Geneva at the lights of Evian on the other side.

The laboratory – a long working day

Erika's predecessor, Heidi Herzog, stayed on for a few weeks to help her to learn the ropes in the laboratory she was to be responsible for. Afterwards, Erika was on her own with one assistant: an older African man called Jim. He did all the cleaning work with the utmost care; he washed out the urine sample containers, centrifuge tubes, and test tubes, and kept everything organised. Erika and Jim could only communicate with each other in one language, English, and neither of them spoke it well. Indeed, Erika had been very bad at English in school. But together, the two of them gradually learned.

Barely two months after Erika's arrival in Elim, a young white doctor offered to help her with the X-rays. Erika was grateful to have a few more hours for the laboratory work, so she showed him everything he needed to know and left him to it. She also asked him to save the yellow and black paper that was used to separate the pieces of X-ray film, instead of throwing it away. It was an excellent resource for handicraft projects for the long-term patients. Once the doctor had left, Jim went to clean the X-ray room – but immediately came back to Erika most upset. He didn't know where to begin – all the sheets of paper were strewn on the floor in complete disorder! Erika forbade him to do any cleaning up, and called the doctor, telling him please to come to the laboratory at once. The doctor appeared, full of anticipation, only to receive an unexpected rebuke from Erika. He did go and clean up. It took a lot of courage for Erika to criticise him so frankly, and she was glad he didn't take it the wrong way. She observes:

> This incident was typical of the sort of "master/servant" attitude that was typical of white South Africans. The "boy" or the "nanny" was expected kindly to clean up the mess, even if the "servant" was an old man, like my Jim, and the "master" a greenhorn, like this young doctor.

Erika's first newsletter from May 16th 1953 vividly describes her first impressions when she looked out of her laboratory window:

> My laboratory is right beside the path between the African hospital and the store, which was the great centre of activity for Africans from Elim and its environs. Each day, those patients who are not bedridden make their way there to buy goods from the inexhaustible riches of the Indian shopkeeper, and, of course, to chat. So, day after day, I can watch this coming and going from my laboratory window. The women's clothing is often very beautiful. There are Tsonga people in their wide skirts, richly decorated with beads, which swing in rhythm with their upright, elastic gait; their shapely, brown shoulders shining in the sunlight. Or Venda women, thin and tall, with finer facial features than the other tribes, dressed in a simple blue-and-red-striped wrap. If a woman has a child, she carries it tied onto her back in a blanket. The treasured purchase is carried atop the customer's head, naturally, whether it is a bottle, a paper bag, or a heavy basket. There are also women in European clothing, sometimes new and sometimes old. The men are all dressed like Europeans, but their clothing is often rather the worse for wear. Sometimes, the people in shabby European clothes strike me as a sort of caricature of the current "native problem". They have lost their self-respect as a result of domination by Europeans.

The working day was long, lasting from seven o'clock in the morning until usually about ten o'clock at night, and Erika had to push herself to become accustomed to it. It is hardly surprising that in her first letters to friends, she repeatedly wrote about her exhaustion. Her main responsibilities in the lab largely consisted of routine tasks. In addition to the examinations that were common in Europe, she tested patients' urine for bilharzia (schistosomiasis), sputum for tuberculosis, stool samples for intestinal schistosomiasis and other parasites, and blood samples for malaria and syphilis. She eventually began to carry out a wider range of tests on her own initiative, making the routine work a bit more tolerable and interesting in the long run. She occasionally made curious discoveries, for example once when she observed fuzzy protozoans shaped like little bears under her microscope. At such times she was grateful for her reference books.

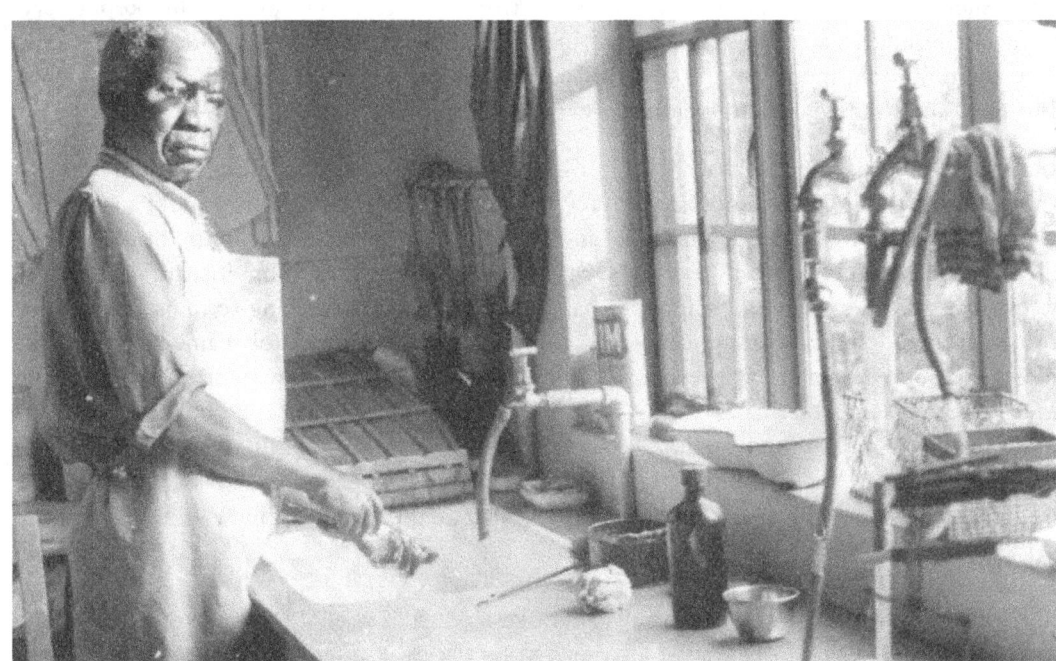

Jim cleaning laboratory utensils, 1953

X-rays were done on Thursday afternoons as needed. Many African patients were transported on stretchers from the African hospital to the X-ray station in the European hospital. Man or woman? It wasn't always easy for Erika to distinguish, because they were covered up to the neck with a light blanket, leaving only their heads and a little curly hair exposed. Rarely was a beard visible. One day, a patient with an extremely enlarged abdomen was brought to her on a stretcher, and she said to the stretcher-bearer, Esrom, "Let's take this maternity case first." Laughter erupted – it was a man!

Esrom was a Jack-of-all-trades and a respected hospital employee, but one day Erika had to criticise him for a mishap. To which he replied, "Thank you, doctor." The Africans courteously thanked everyone for everything. On another occasion, she had to make a number of X-rays of an Indian patient. At the end he thanked her, saying that now he felt a lot better.

African laboratory technicians: why not?

Erika was alone in the laboratory when she started work in Elim. At one point, another doctor joined her to help out for a short time, and he immediately remarked that there was really too much work for one person to handle. "It was truly a struggle, but there simply wasn't enough money for two technicians", Erika remembers. Then it happened that one of Marie-

Louise Martin's students from Lemana was sent to Elim as a patient. Marie-Louise said to Erika, "Please look after my Julius!" A blood test showed an extremely low haemoglobin level, so Erika asked for a stool sample. Julius was found to be infected with schistosomiasis, and oesophageal varices had developed. These "varicose veins in the oesophagus" can sometimes lead to vomiting of blood. Despite his illness, Julius wrote his matriculation examinations. But he was not successful, and he decided to go to work in a mine. Erika wanted to prevent this, and asked her boss, Dr Rosset, whether she could train Julius to work in the lab. "Africans aren't capable of doing things like that", was his initial response, but he agreed to give it a try. Erika recalls:

> Julius was thrilled! He read all the books that I had in the lab., and even made suggestions as to different tests to try out; in short, he was talented, motivated, and creative. Working with him was a complete success. But then the bleeding from the oesophagus became more frequent. We sent him to Pretoria for bypass surgery, but the night before the operation was scheduled he began bleeding uncontrollably and died.
>
> I went looking for his relatives to tell them the sad news, in the company of Marie Tinguely, who was the head of household services. The family lived far away, deep in the bush, in a little village that could only be reached by means of a long journey on foot. No sooner had we given them the news of Julius's death, than they were gripped by intense grief and the women began to weep aloud and cry out. It was the first time I had witnessed such ritual mourning. I sat there helpless, not knowing what to say. The family had pinned its hopes on Julius. Luckily, he wasn't their only son. His younger brother later succeeded in graduating from High School, and we heard that he had even become a teacher.

By demonstrating so clearly that he was capable of becoming an expert technician, Julius blazed a path for other Africans to be trained in the laboratory. The next to join Erika was Samuel Kumalo, the son of a chief. He had completed the High School course in Lemana and had to find a job to bridge the long waiting period before he assumed his father's functions. He also worked well with Erika, as well as with her successor. All the African technicians became dependable colleagues. There were not yet any recognised diplomas for technicians in the 1950s, but as far as Erika remembers, their pay was on the same level as that of the nurses.

Nationalisation of the schools: the spread of "Bantu Education"

After the National Party came to power in 1948, the ideological control of the curriculum of schools became an important part of apartheid policy, and was pushed forward with the enactment of a series of laws. When Erika began working in Elim in 1952, the primary schools had just been affected. The main goal of "Bantu Education" was to impart just enough knowledge to the children to enable them to be good workers in the future – but under no circumstances should they glimpse "the green pastures of the Whites". So English disappeared from the primary schools, and for the first six years the children were taught in the local vernacular language. At the next level they were suddenly confronted with learning English and Afrikaans simultaneously, which was too great a burden for most of them. The new regulations had drastic effects on the mission schools.

In 1956, the secondary schools and high schools were also subjected to the "Bantu education" policy, and one by one, the Swiss teachers hired by the mission had to be replaced by South African teachers – preferably Afrikaners. The higher classes in Lemana, which were preparing students for the matriculation certificate that was required for university entrance, were among the last to be affected. When it happened, half of the subjects were taught in English, and the other half in Afrikaans – but things were occasionally switched around depending on the situation. All this led to total confusion. Students throughout South Africa who wanted to go to a University were very disadvantaged, because they had to begin by catching up on their English. "It's no coincidence that a series of revolts began in the schools, culminating in the student uprising in Soweto in 1976," says Erika. She saw the results of the changes very clearly in the hospital:

> When I was first in Elim, it was possible to converse with students from the top classes in Lemana in English. But later, up to the time when I left, this was no longer the case, since their English skills were so poor.

A new challenge: Medical School in Johannesburg

During her four years in the laboratory, Erika spent several relaxing holidays at another mission station, in Masana, since she obviously couldn't afford a hotel vacation on her missionary salary. She hiked with enthusiasm in the beautiful landscape, and got along well with the Medical Superintendent there, Dr Alwin Beugger, and his wife, Louisli. Erika recalls:

> It must have been 1955 when Dr Beugger turned to me one day and said that if I had been in his hospital, he would have sent me to medical school long ago. Spending a lifetime working in the lab. didn't suit me, he thought. He himself had begun as a male nurse in Shiluvane, and then the mission had sent him to Johannesburg to study medicine. He had later expanded the Health Point in Masana into a hospital.
>
> I turned his idea over in my mind, but didn't speak to anyone about it except my best friend Eveline Jacot, the secretary in Elim. I didn't want all sorts of people giving me advice, preferring instead to decide for myself whether this was right for me. I finally came to the conclusion: yes, indeed, this is my path. I then spoke with Dr Rosset, our Superintendent. He was initially very sceptical about whether this made sense, in view of my age, but he eventually agreed. My studies could be financed in advance out of the Hospital's "Leave-and-Loan" fund, into which we paid the difference between the higher salary we were paid by the State and the lower mission salary to which we were entitled. I would eventually have to pay back the cost of my studies by the same method.
>
> Since everything was still very uncertain and I wanted to avoid Elim's village gossip, I continued to keep my plans secret. So I was very pleased that on the very same date that I had been asked to come to Johannesburg for a preliminary interview, I was invited by a retired missionary couple living there, René Cuenot and his wife, to join them for a concert by a Swiss harpsichord player. They knew that I loved ancient music and had already got permission from Dr Rosset to invite me. So I was able to travel to Johannesburg without anyone knowing what else I planned to do there.

While she was in Johannesburg, Erika happened to bump into Gertie Friede, a nurse who had been working in Elim not long before. She was the daughter of Jewish immigrants. Erika shared her study plans with her, and told her she was hoping to find a place to live with an English-speaking family. Gertie telephoned almost immediately afterwards, and said that her parents in Johannesburg would be happy to host Erika until she found a suitable family. The Friedes' house in Emmarentia, a suburb of Johannesburg, finally became Erika's home for her entire study period. She was welcomed like a daughter – with all the advantages and none of the obligations, as she puts it. She is still in touch with the Friedes' daughter Gertie.

Everything had come together perfectly. Erika was also lucky that she was not forced to take the matriculation examination for university entrance. That might have happened, as the Swiss Matura was not recognised in South Africa. But the university accepted Erika's doctorate in botany as proof that she was qualified to enter the university, and she was even given credit for her courses in botany, zoology, and physics in Basel, so she only had to make up chemistry, which she could do in four months rather than a year.

Back in Elim, Erika managed to press ahead with her final preparations for study. She found a laboratory technician from Basel, Elisabeth Meister, who continued her work. And in the few remaining weeks before her departure, Erika went to a farm in Bandolierkop, near Elim, where she took intensive English lessons from farm owner Edmond Thomas's English wife, Auntie Pat, who had been an English teacher in Lemana.

Johannesburg – a new world

Her studies began just two months after the first visit to Johannesburg, in autumn 1956, at the University of the Witwatersrand, commonly known as "Wits". Five years and four months of extremely rigorous study were in store for Erika. But at the beginning there was also a new world that opened itself up to her; city life in Johannesburg. She was very fortunate that she could live with Grethe and Heinrich Friede, whose two children had already left the nest. When she arrived, she realised that she scarcely had clothes for life in the city – in recent years, her laboratory overalls had been all she needed. Grethe Friede had a remedy. She was actually in the middle of doing a sewing course, and could show Erika how to sew very attractive clothes. Erika's own mother had been very discouraging – after one failed attempt when she was an adolescent she told her she would never learn! Nevertheless, Erika had once created a lovely bathing suit – knitted it, in fact! And if she had really lacked manual dexterity, what would have become of her later when she had to sew wounds in the emergency room or perform eye surgery?

Early in the morning, Erika could often get a lift with Heinrich Friede into the city and to the university. In the evenings, after she returned home, she and the Friedes would take the two dogs for their obligatory walk up the Melville Koppies, a ridge almost right beside the house, which had been declared a nature reserve thanks to the Friedes' efforts. Archaeological finds

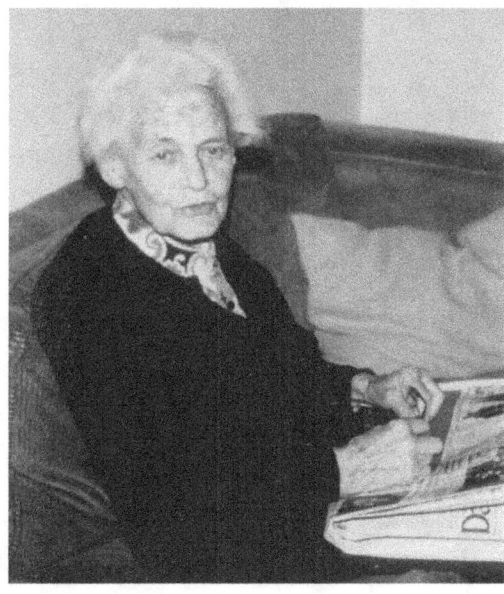
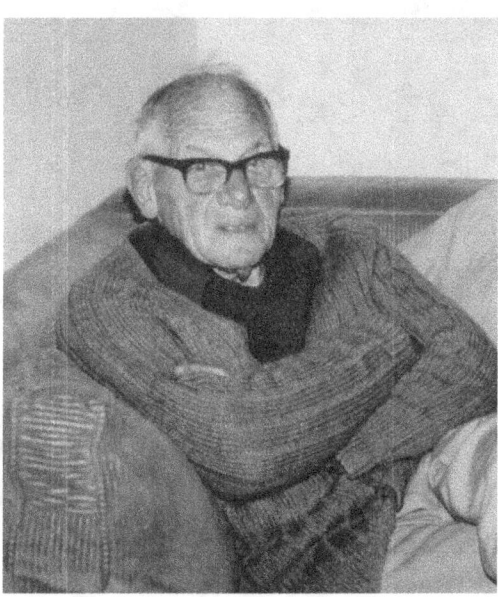

Erika's hosts during her studies in Johannesburg, Greta and Heinrich Friede, 1961

were eventually uncovered on the Koppies, among them an iron-smelting furnace. At weekends, they often went for hikes together with other friends.

Erika discovered that she and her hosts had many interests in common. The Friedes were members of the *Bird Society* and the *Tree Society*, among other things. Heavyset and rather slow-moving, Heinrich was somewhat fonder of the *Tree Society*, as the birds had commonly long since flown away before he had a chance to set eyes on them. Erika occasionally went with Grethe by car to a concert in the city. The public buses did not run after 7 p.m., and after that it was dangerous to be out and about alone. Through the Friedes, Erika had her first real contact with the world of Jewish tradition. In Johannesburg, there was a very large Jewish population. Many of them were intellectuals – practically half of the doctors and many of Erika's fellow students were Jewish.

In Johannesburg Erika saw apartheid with new eyes. In contrast to rural Elim, where as a European she could move quite freely among the Africans and work with them, the racial segregation here was much more visible and was characterised by mutual distrust. Erika encountered apartheid at every step. She saw African domestic workers sitting on the grass verges beside the road, since they could not find anywhere else to relax – the park benches were labelled "Europeans only".

No seats for Africans!

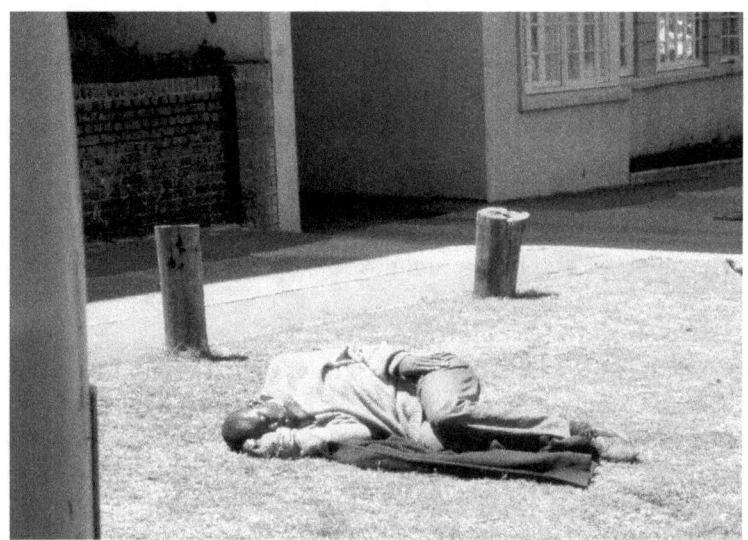

Almost forty and a University student!

Erika's studies began in September 1956. During the four-month chemistry practical course in her first year, she was assigned to a supervisor who turned out to be a friend of Mrs Thurneysen, the wife of Rev. Thurneysen in Basel. The chemistry lecturer, Professor Isaacs, was very kind to Erika and followed her progress with interest. By the time of her graduation ceremony he had become the Rector of the University, and he offered his congratulations: "Well done!"

The chemistry course was followed by anatomy and physiology in the second year. At the start, all of the students had to fill in their current age on a list. It was the June 1st, so Erika could still write "39 years," which was so much younger than forty – her 40th birthday was on June 14th. She was looking forward to her first lecture with Professor Dart, a palaeoanthropologist who had discovered an important link between humans and apes in South Africa. However, he did not begin by lecturing the class about his area of expertise, as she had expected, but instead drew a curve on the blackboard that illustrated the development of human learning capacity. According to the knowledge of the day, an individual's capacity to learn increased from birth onwards, peaking at age twenty – the age of Erika's fellow students – and reaching its low point at age forty: quite dispiriting!

At the beginning of the second year of study, the students were divided up into groups of six, who worked together at the dissecting tables and often remained together for the rest of their studies, including periods of practical work in various hospital departments. In the group Erika joined, most of the students, like her, were older and already had a profession, except for a young Jewish woman, Judy Issroff. Erika became friends with her, and also with Monica Simon, whom she described colourfully:

> Monica was a chain smoker. I too smoked every once in a while, but Monica had to leave the dissecting room and go outside every twenty minutes to smoke one, otherwise she couldn't stand it. She was married and had no children. So she decided she would pursue a satisfying career and began medical school. In her sixth year of study, she got pregnant and had to stop, as she was no longer allowed to be around patients once she reached her sixth month of pregnancy. So she stopped studying and gave birth to a boy, a prematurely born smoker's child, all skin and bones. He developed healthily though, and once he was three years old, she resumed her studies. But then she got pregnant again and gave up. I spent a lot of time with her family when the Friedes were on holiday. Monica's father was very musical and he had a large record collection. They were Russian Jews, and Monica's mother, who was not very fluent in English, used to speak Russian at the table, too. Monica and I worked very well together when revising our lecture notes.

For dissection, each group of students was allocated an entire human body, not just limbs as was done in Switzerland. "Indeed, there were enough unknown Africans dying in the city," Erika added by way of explanation, going on to say:

> Before we performed our first dissection, the university pastor held a funeral service. I was very impressed, and found it striking and beautiful. Thus we honoured the deceased and showed them respect. We were also offered psychiatric support for the tough anatomy year, and the assistants were trained to support us and to notice when one of us wasn't doing well. In that way, anatomy was actually the most humane department.

The third year of training, beginning in the autumn of 1958, covered pathology and public health and was less rigorous than the others. So Erika suggested to her mother that it would be a good time to visit her in South Africa. Her mother gladly accepted the invitation.

Erika recalls:

> My mother was seventy-two years old at the time, and she was thrilled by her six-month visit to Africa, the first major journey of her life. She was warmly received all around, especially by the nurses in Elim. When I was at the university in Johannesburg, she was able to stay with friends. During my vacation, we took trips to other mission stations and to Victoria Falls. She was particularly impressed by the missionary work in Shiluvane.

Apartheid within the universities

By Erika's fourth year of studies, 1959, the apartheid government had already been in power for eleven years. Little by little, various legal changes came into force that were intended to keep the Africans "on the other side of the fence". The universities were also affected. In the University of Natal the medical school was for Indian, coloured and African students. In Pretoria there was a substantial medical school for whites only, with mostly Afrikaans-speaking students. In the Cape Province there were the University of Cape Town; the University of the Western Cape for "coloureds" (people of mixed race), with no Faculty of Medicine; and the European university in Stellenbosch mainly for Afrikaans-speakers, with the Theological Faculty of the Dutch Reformed Church. Later, the University of the North for Africans only was established near Pietersburg. In Johannesburg, in addition to the purely European Rand Afrikaans University, with no Faculty of Medicine, there was the multiracial University of the Witwatersrand, "Wits", where Erika was studying. During Erika's years there, the university was faced with the problem of whether it could remain multiracial. Erika's class was very mixed; of the 20% of the students who were not Jewish or white, about equal numbers were African, or of mixed race, Indian, or Chinese.

Racial discrimination manifested itself in everyday student life:

> For example, in the pathology courses, European students could be present for the autopsies of all corpses, but African students could only be present when the deceased was non-European, meaning that they had far less illustrative material compared to the others.

> At one point, a call went up to organise a protest march against racial segregation at the universities. Most of us participated, myself included, of course. Back then, it was still possible to have a student protest march without the police reacting with violence. On the day of the protest, the "Black Sash" women picketed in front of the university. The Black Sash was an organisation of European women founded in the Cape Province in 1955, when the National Party stripped away the voting rights of people of mixed race. These women protested against the action and demonstrated in front of the Parliament building wearing black sashes – giving the movement its name. They also opened a legal aid office for Africans in Johannesburg and protested against the forced relocation of Africans in the late 1960s and early 1970s.

This too was an impressive experience for Erika, witnessing Europeans in Johannesburg expressing their solidarity and protesting against the growing discrimination against Africans in the apartheid system.

The final three years of study consisted of hands-on training and were extremely challenging for Erika. "Had I known what was in store for me, I probably wouldn't have had the courage to do it", she observes in retrospect. In surgery and in medicine, the students often had to work seven days a week. After the 5 p.m. lectures work in the wards started immediately and went on until midnight or later. One advantage of the system was that it gave the students a head start in practical experience compared with medical students in Switzerland. For example they learned what to do during the acute phase of a heart attack when a patient was admitted at night, rather than only seeing such patients the next morning when they were doing somewhat better, as would have been the case in Switzerland. They also participated actively in all examinations. However, it was hard to stay awake in afternoon lectures after the long nights and mornings in the hospital ward.

The practical training in surgery took place in both African and European hospitals. Together with colleagues from her working group, Erika rented a room near the hospital in Johannesburg, since there was no way of getting home at night. One of Erika's reminiscences concerns an incident involving the Prime Minister:

Once, during the Rand Easter Show (a major agricultural exhibition in Johannesburg), Prime Minister Verwoerd was shot. He was brought in as an emergency case to the European hospital, where we happened to be on duty. One of our students got ready to examine the patient, who had a gunshot wound in the head. Just as he was about to begin, the Registrar came in and asked him if he knew who the patient was. He responded, "Oh, it's just another drunkard!" He was then set right and prevented from touching the Prime Minister again. The Prime Minister was immediately transferred to Pretoria, where he would be much more at home than in the multicultural city of Johannesburg, which the National Government abhorred.

In the final academic year, the main focus was on gynaecology and obstetrics. It encompassed five weeks of practical training in the maternity ward of the three-thousand-bed Baragwanath Hospital (now the Chris Hani Baragwanath Hospital) in Soweto, where Erika gained lots of practical experience – conducting fifty births, for example – as well as a final month spent in the large Alexandra Township clinic. It was the last year when that was possible; from then on, the university authorities felt that in a climate of increasing tension the risk for the students was too high. Erika has fond memories of this period:

> We four students were housed in the clinic itself, and were responsible for everything. The doctors made rounds in the morning, but we were on our own in the afternoon and at night. The next hospital was quite a distance away. In an emergency we could call someone there for help, but we handled a lot on our own. We made lots of home visits in the township during the day, but – beginning with the class of our year – we were no longer allowed to conduct home births at night, since it would have been too dangerous for us. Evidently, I was greatly appreciated during the home visits, as I learned from Mrs. Friede, who did voluntary work as a pharmacist in Alexandra. It was probably because I was more mature than my classmates and was comfortable around Africans from my time in Elim. Their appreciation for me was also revealed when, six months later, I was the only one of the former students to be invited to the Christmas celebration in Alexandra. The entire community was there. I remember how a brass band played, and a tiny little girl stood up and began conducting it. I asked her mother how old she was – one-and-a-half years! And the rhythm was already in her.

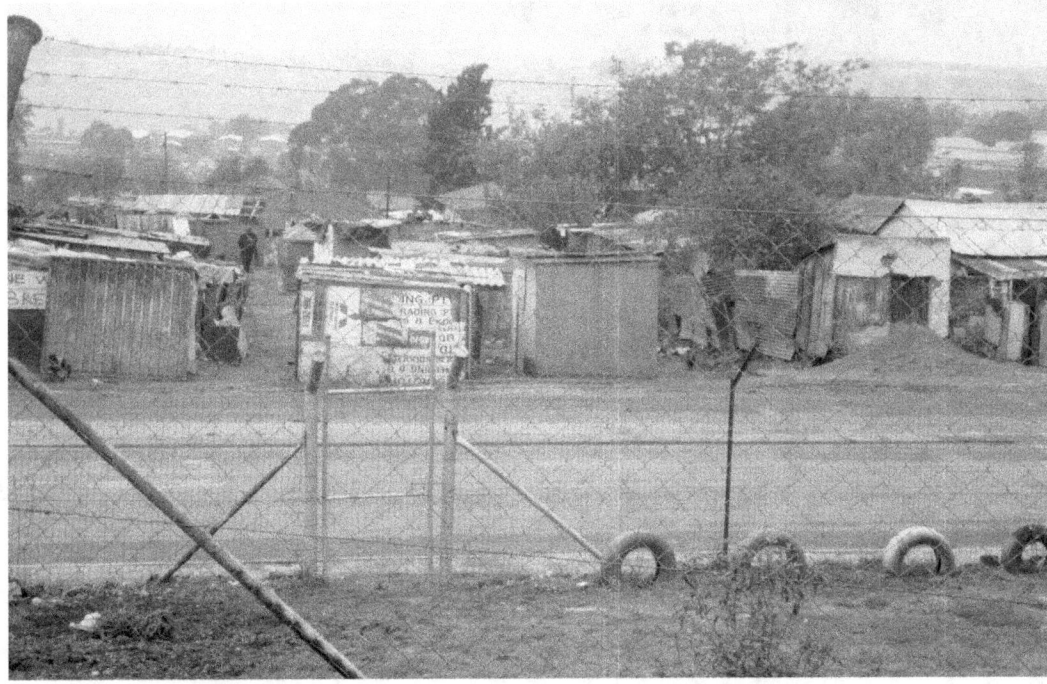

Alexandra Township, 1961

The time in Alexandra opened many of my fellow-students' eyes to the living conditions of the Africans. Most people living in Johannesburg had scarcely ever set eyes on the townships and had no idea how the people there really lived. A maid would go home at night and her employer would have no clue about her family, her problems, and all the work she would have to get done in her own home before returning the next day to take care of her employer's household.

The year of residency

After successfully passing the final State examinations, Erika had to spend a year as a resident House Officer in a hospital so that she could complete the requirements for registration as a doctor and be entitled to practise medicine. The Elim Superintendent, Dr Rosset, recommended that she should do this before she went on leave to Switzerland, so she spent the year 1961–2 in the Baragwanath Hospital in Soweto. Erika said:

> I could have completed my residency in Elim, but I thought it wiser to make my first mistakes elsewhere, not in the place where I wanted to stay! In my first half year, in the surgical department, I saw and treated virtually the whole spectrum of diseases. I was on duty almost every other night. It was extremely tough, but I had a good boss. Almost all the doctors were Jewish. It impressed me how fully dedicated to the patients they were. At times, it was anything but amusing the way that patients would be brought in, drunk and bleeding. The awful mixture of smells – alcohol and blood! You just had to endure it, even when it almost made you sick. I completed the second half of my residency year in the department of medicine, which suited me better than surgery. It was much more personal, allowing for interaction with patients.

Graduation 1961. On the steps of Wits University

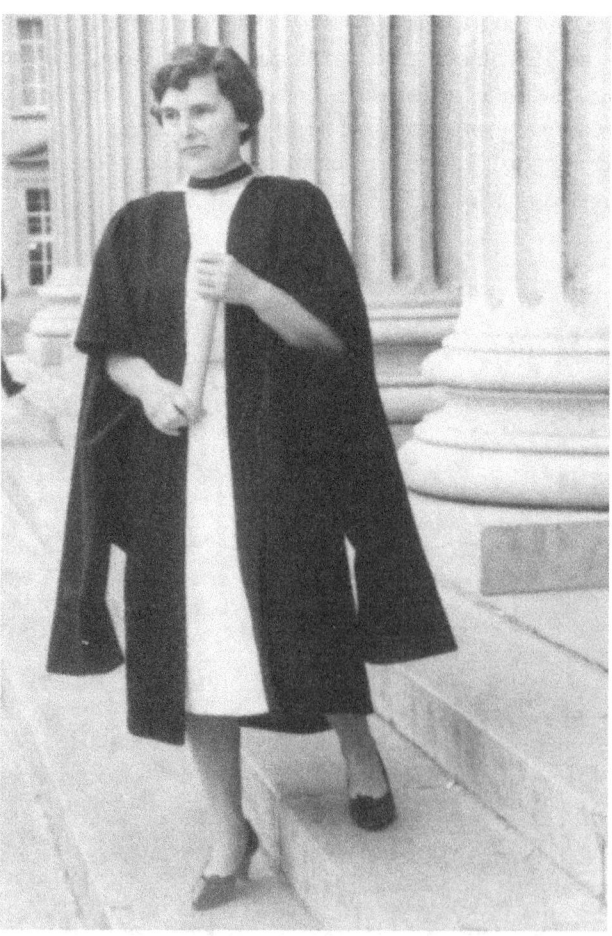

Erika remembers one night when she was on call for another department and was sent for to look at a patient with pancreatitis, who had fallen into a coma:

> On my way there I thought about what I should do. I was alone and would have to decide myself. First, I went over the patient's medical history and discovered he was also diabetic. My conclusion was that he had fallen into a diabetic coma, which didn't necessarily have anything to do with the pancreatitis. So I gave him a shot of glucose. In the case of a diabetic coma, where you don't know if it's due to hypo- or hyperglycaemia, you can always administer a shot of glucose. It never hurts, and it works immediately if it is hypoglycaemia. And that was exactly what happened. Before I was through with the injection, the patient sat up and laughed. All the forty men in the room laughed too, and thought I was a doctor with magical powers. I was incredibly proud that everything had turned out so well.

> Overall, my year of residency was a very instructive experience. It really prepared us well to practise medicine. I became aware of this later in Elim. When young doctors came to us from Switzerland, they had more theoretical knowledge, but they knew much less about what to do in the clinical situation, and had fewer practical skills.

During her residency period, Erika had a visitor from Switzerland, Martin Schwarz, a friend of her brother's. He and his sister Marianne were the children of Rev. Schwarz, with whom Erika's sister Trudi had worked so many years ago on the "Ulme" social project. The Schwarz family had all become active in the Swiss anti-apartheid movement. Martin arrived shortly after the massacre at Sharpeville, the event that triggered the abandonment of non-violent resistance by the ANC (African National Congress) in South Africa. Erika was able to give Martin some insight into what had been happening in South Africa, and in return she heard the latest news about the anti-apartheid movement in Switzerland. When she retired and returned home in 1984 she was also active against apartheid.

At last, a vacation!

Following the successful completion of her studies and residency, and after ten years of service in South Africa, the Mission granted Erika a year of paid leave. In February 1962, she and two colleagues headed home by way of Venice, travelling the length of the East coast of Africa in an Italian ship.

Specializing in ophthalmology

During her hard-earned time off back home in Basel, Erika began looking around for opportunities to continue training in gynaecology and obstetrics, which she believed would be important for her future work as a doctor in Elim. She enquired about a six-month practical work placement in Obstetrics in the Basel Women's Hospital. The people who interviewed her considered this to be very short – but were amazed when they asked how many births she had observed, and Erika said she had conducted more than fifty births herself.

However, a letter then arrived from Elim that opened up a whole new perspective: Erika was asked if she would like to take over the Elim eye hospital. If she agreed, the Superintendent, Dr J. Rosset, and his wife, Dr Odette Rosset, who was the head of the Eye Hospital, recommended that she should "orient herself a bit" for one or two months before her urgently awaited return to Elim. Erika thought about working in ophthalmology. Why not? Eyes are a fine speciality for a woman – but the idea had simply never occurred to her before. After careful consideration, she decided to say "yes".

However, the demand from Elim that she should not only learn a new speciality but come back to South Africa in a few months put her under a great deal of pressure. And she had other doubts, because she foresaw major problems when she got there. The outgoing head of the eye hospital, Dr Odette Rosset, was a rather difficult individual. She had built up the eye hospital herself. She had begun with only rudimentary specialist knowledge, but had eventually become an accomplished surgeon. Now she wanted to retire along with her husband – and as soon as possible. She wanted Erika to come as her replacement almost immediately, regardless of how well she was prepared for the new position, so she could introduce her quickly and then leave.

Erika held her ground, however, and insisted on a thorough training. She rejected the notion that lesser qualifications should suffice for African patients. A German colleague suggested that she could fill in for Erika in Elim while she completed her training, but Dr Rosset found this unacceptable, and opted to stay longer herself, still intending to show Erika the ropes personally. It was a very stressful time of tough negotiations with the hospital and the Mission. Erika even wondered whether she should join a different mission, and went so far as to discuss the possibility with the president of the Basel Mission, Dr Jacques Rossel.

Erika's specialist training began with a year working under Professor Rintelen at the Basel Eye Hospital. The first thing he did was to give Erika a copy of his own textbook, *Lehrbuch für Augenheilkunde* (Fundamentals of Ophthalmology). In the course of her thorough study of this standard reference text, she realised that though she had qualified as a doctor in South Africa she still had a lot to learn. The Swiss medical students had learned a lot more about the "minor" subjects, especially ophthalmology and dermatology. Eventually, she worked in the outpatients' department of the Eye Hospital, and later on the private and men's wards.

After that, she completed a six-month diploma course in London. Her feelings of depression and self-doubt returned, making her studies especially difficult. Nevertheless, she made it to the final examination for the Diploma in Ophthalmology. She had few illusions about her chances, knowing that no more than forty percent of the candidates ever passed. After the last exam, everyone had to wait in a special room to receive the results. At last, someone appeared

At the Basel Eye Hospital

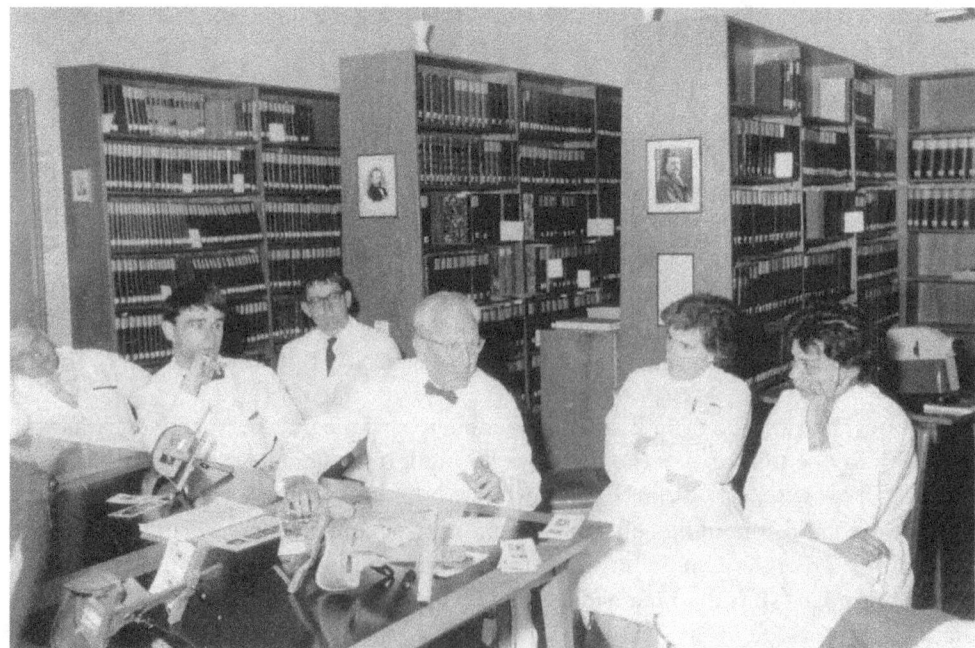

in the doorway, calling out numbers and announcing: "Sorry, you failed" or "Congratulations, you passed." When Erika's number came up, she could scarcely believe that she had passed. She had rather given up hope, because she had made a silly mistake in one answer.

After that, she had three months to practise surgical procedures in the Basel Eye Hospital. Her colleagues were all preparing to obtain the Swiss qualification for medical specialists, recognition by the *Foederatio Medicorum Helveticorum* (FMH), for which they must conduct at least four cataract operations in their fourth year of specialist training, under the supervision of a senior physician. Since they were only allowed to operate on the second eye of a patient whose first eye had been successfully operated on by the Professor, there were only a few suitable patients, who had to be shared among the students. That made it all the more surprising that all of Erika's colleagues generously gave her first priority, so that she was able to operate on twelve cataracts within the three months. They said, "This is our contribution to *Brot für Alle*." ("Bread for All" is a Swiss Church NGO working on development.) Erika remains deeply moved by the gesture to this day. She spent long hours preparing for the operations, practising on pigs' eyes until late at night, with a lot of help from the ophthalmic surgeon Peter Huber.

In the meantime, Erika's tough negotiations with Elim Hospital, the Moderator of the Evangelical Presbyterian Church of South Africa (EPCSA), and the general secretary of the *Département Missionnaire* in Lausanne, had finally been resolved. Dr and Mrs. Rosset had left Elim, leaving the path clear for Erika to return and take up her position under the new Superintendent, Dr Pierre Jaques. Sadly, she was preceded by rumours spread by Dr Odette Rosset that she was "a bit of a *Résistante*" – a difficult person. As a result, Dr Jaques initially behaved cautiously towards Erika. But he soon realised that she was not really difficult, and they worked well together. At her request, Erika was granted her own little house. She began to build up her influence within the Eye Hospital and open up new possibilities.

VI Head of the Eye Hospital in Elim

Returning to Elim as a doctor

In the summer of 1965, Erika returned to Elim as a fully-qualified ophthalmologist. By this time her predecessor, Dr Odette Rosset, had already been gone for a month. Sister Helen, who was totally accustomed to Dr Rosset's working methods after more than thirty years with her, welcomed Erika and took her on her first rounds of the hospital. The day remains vivid in Erika's memory. Inspectors from the South African Nursing Council were also there, conducting a routine inspection of the nursing school, accompanied by the matron, Gabrielle Guy. And just by chance, Erika overheard a question directed to the matron by one of the inspectors: "Why don't you have a school for ophthalmic nursing here?" Erika commented later:

> Looking back, I see that coincidence as God's guidance. I kept that remark at the back of my mind until I finally had the opportunity to make the school a reality ten years later!

Apart from this, Erika's first day back in Elim was exhausting. Many patients were waiting for cataract operations, and every case had complications, as the damage to the eyes was further compounded by trachoma or other infections. In her first three months, Erika conducted seventy-five cataract operations! She structured her daily routine, operating on two days of the week. On the first day, she handled the non-infected cases of cataracts and, later, glaucoma. Glaucoma was previously only treated with eye drops, not surgically, as no effective method was known. On the second operating day she mainly treated trachoma, which involved surgery for entropion, the condition in which the upper eyelid has been deformed by scarring, and the eyelashes rub against the cornea, which leads to blindness. Entropion is the result of many years of infection. At the hospital, they usually saw trachoma cases only after the damage had been done. Entropion can be corrected by a relatively simple operation, arrived at after testing more complex methods, which works so well that relapses are rare. The eye diseases that Erika encountered covered the whole range familiar to her from Switzerland. The only one she did not see among her African patients was retinal detachment. But there were a marked number of cases of pterygium, a fan-shaped growth of the conjunctiva over the cornea, as well as the common allergic eye disease called "spring catarrh".

Left:
Signpost to eye consultations

Right:
Erika operating on an eye, assisted by Nurse Stephina and Sister Ida Schmidlin

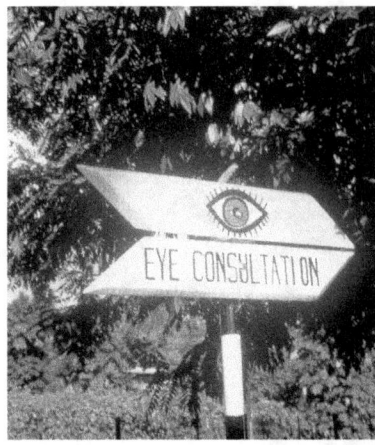
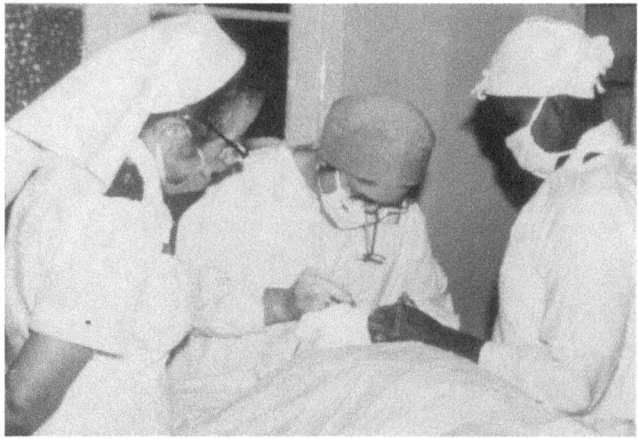

Erika was the only doctor in the eye hospital, and was thus essentially on duty or on call every day and every night, but luckily she was seldom called in for emergency cases at night. She had to go for long periods without a vacation, and often felt alone with her responsibilities. She also missed interacting with expert colleagues, as she wrote in her first report to her ophthalmology professor, Prof. Rintelen, in Basel. His original recommendation, that she should refer difficult cases to bigger hospitals in Pretoria or Johannesburg, proved to be unrealistic, because the patients were unwilling to leave their familiar environment. It was not a question of cost, because a patient only had to pay one rand for every hospital visit, whether for an outpatient consultation or a longer stay. So Erika did whatever was in her power to best help her patients. Time and time again she asked herself the same question, "Should I do nothing, since I don't have the proper training? Then the patient will go blind. Or should I do my best, taking a chance to try and save an eye?" Sometimes she could take a patient to Johannesburg, operate on him with another doctor, and take him back again. She also had the opportunity to participate in the regular refresher courses for local ophthalmologists given on Saturday mornings by Professor Luntz of the Johannesburg Medical School, which was a great help for her practice in Elim.

In the first few years, Erika's main concern was to practise the best possible curative ophthalmology, just as she had learned it in Switzerland. It was precisely this high aspiration that repeatedly led to conflicts between Erika and her closest colleague, Sister Helen, who was a deaconess from Lausanne:

> Helen was completely exasperated by me. She had come to Elim with Dr Rosset thirty years before, when the Eye Hospital was founded. Everything had been much simpler in those days. There had never been so many different diagnoses, and everything had worked without any of this new "fancy business". She rejected all my suggestions for improvements, but with time I realised that I just had to mention an improvement once and then stop talking about it. If I did that, she herself would eventually make the same suggestion. In this way, I was finally able to introduce some changes. I liked Helen, actually, and had even spent my vacation with her when I worked in the lab. It was just difficult for her to adjust to a new doctor after so many years with another.

However, there was another problem; driving. Erika was dependent on Sister Helen for rides, as there was no public transportation for Europeans. She was not very adept at driving, but drove at breakneck speed anyway, and Erika was always thankful when she arrived in one piece. So she decided to learn to drive, to give herself some independence and enable her to take visitors around.

After about two years, Sister Helen gave up working in Elim and went to work in Morija (Lesotho), in a hospital belonging to the Paris Mission. Her successor, likewise a senior European nurse from Switzerland, also had difficulties, due to her lack of leadership skills and her insufficient knowledge of English, which diminished her in the eyes of the African nurses. Many of them would have been better qualified for such a senior position, but, in the apartheid system, a European nurse was automatically given the superior role.

For the first eight years, Erika was the sole eye specialist for the 60-bed hospital, as well as for another 40 patients, not bedridden, who were treated in the so-called "Village," an adjoining building. Hence, Erika always had about 100 patients to look after. It meant a lot of work, especially when she had to look up and read up about any condition that was new to her in the specialist literature. Did any time remain for private life? Indeed it did!

Her own home with a garden

Until her own little bungalow-style home was completed, Erika lived in the Nurses' Home. To the east, a plot of thornbush savannah on the slope of Elim Hill had been cleared and filled in with earth in preparation for her new home. Within the area specified for the house, she was free to determine the arrangement of the rooms to be built: a living room, a bedroom, a guest room, and the obligatory *stoep*, a wide veranda enclosed with mosquito screens. There was enough land for a garden 30 metres by 30 thirty metres. From the wild bushes and trees on the site, Erika kept two marula trees and her favourite "sickle bush" – which is sometimes also called "Christmas tree", because around Christmas-time it bears beautiful two-coloured flowers, mauve and yellow, that hang from the branches like little lanterns. The house was given the name *Enkoveni*, meaning "on the hillside," and Erika was able to move in early in 1966.

She described her new paradise in glowing terms:

> For my cosy eating area, I was furnished with a table and a corner bench by a carpentry school, and the rest of the furniture was added gradually. In the garden, I put in flowerbeds around the perimeter of the small front lawn, including some lovely trees: a cassia, a poinciana (flamboyant), lemon and grapefruit trees, and an orange tree. Sadly, I was only able to enjoy the oranges the first year, as later they were always stolen. At the bottom of the garden were the vegetable beds and a compost pit, and beside them several poinsettias. In contrast to the potted versions many of us see in Europe at Christmas, in Africa these can grow to more than two metres. Passion fruits grew and thrived on the fence, though I usually had to surrender them to the monkeys, who were much faster than me. At the top of the garden I had a mulberry tree, several papayas, the basis for all fruit dishes, and – unique in Elim! – strawberries. The garage was overgrown with passion flowers, grapes, and bougainvillea. Behind the house was a small chicken farm with five chickens. So I was largely self-sufficient.

Erika's house, Enkoveni, 1962

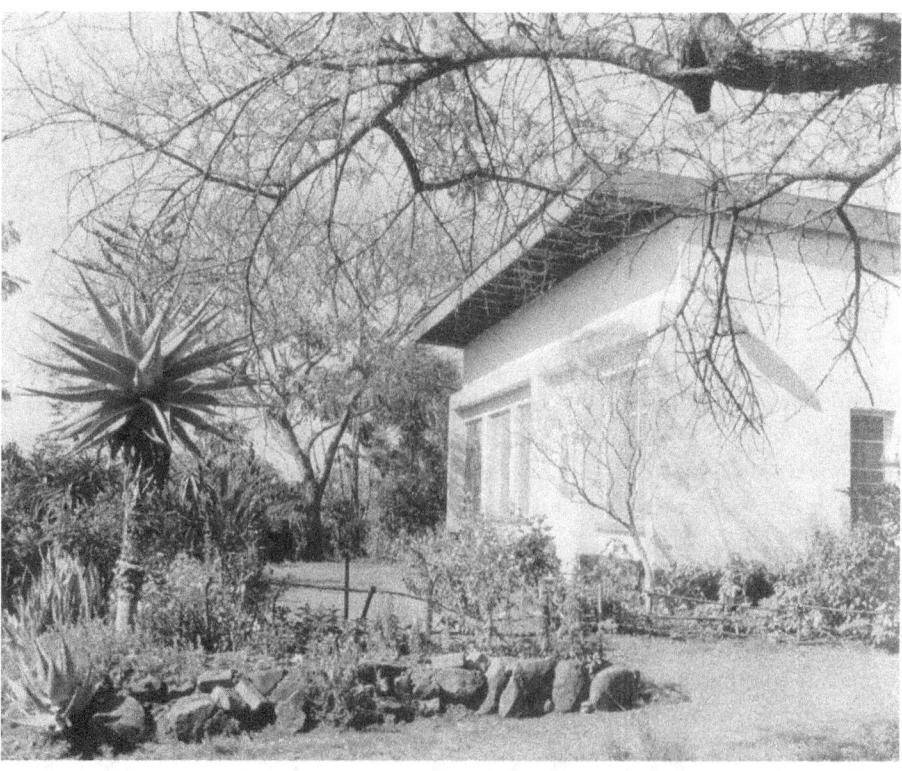

Hilda and Jackson

It all had to be maintained, of course, and I didn't have enough time to do that besides all the work at the hospital. We Europeans were expected to hire someone to look after our house and garden, as the local people desperately needed jobs. And so Hilda Mutenda became my wonderful, trusted housekeeper. For the garden, I initially hired a schoolboy, as was often done. He lived in a little house beside us, and his school fees and books were paid for in return for around two hours of work in the garden each day. We were later joined by Jackson Maluleke, who helped out part time.

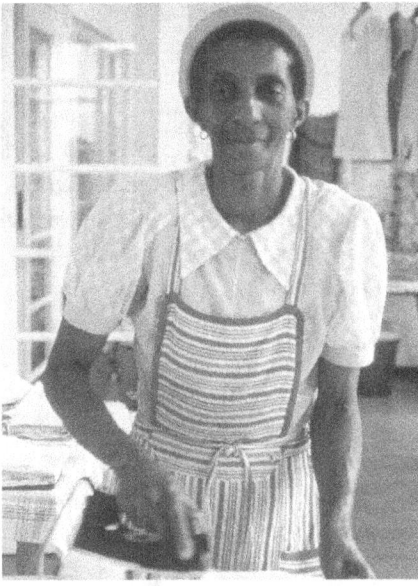
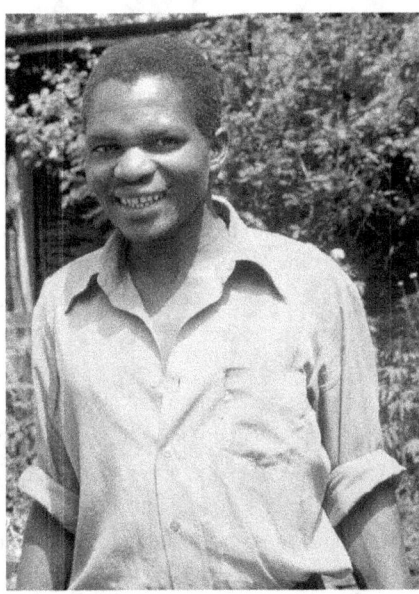

Left:
Hilda

Right:
Jackson

Hilda was my companion for almost the entire eighteen years that I lived in my little house. She was an excellent cook, but I worried about her delicate health and had to make sure that she didn't clean too much. Unlike most of the other Africans, she was a passionate reader, and was always asking for an interesting book. It was very hard for her to say goodbye to me. In a long, moving letter, she told me what I meant to her. She was the only person who regularly wrote to me and told me how she was doing after I returned to Switzerland. Writing letters isn't really part of the Africans' deep-seated oral culture.

Jackson, the gardener, a man with a cheerful disposition, looked after my garden with great devotion. The vegetables were much more important to him than the "useless" flowers, so we weren't allowed to uproot any of the tomatoes that sprang up on their own between the flowers. They were the hardiest plants, anyway. And at the very bottom of the garden, a whole bed of chillies suddenly appeared, a most precious and popular spice that one could even earn money with.

One day, Jackson announced his desire to try his luck in Johannesburg – one of the greatest temptations, but one that usually ended in disappointment. Hilda and I tried to dissuade him, but we also wanted to allow him the freedom to make his own decision. After a couple of months, he came back as thin as a rake, and miserable. Since he could only stay in the city illegally, on account of the apartheid laws, he had slept in cement pipes for building work that were lying by the roadside, and starved his way through. He had worked – illegally – for just a short time, laying tiles. We had to nurse him back to health for a while before he could eat properly again. From then on he stayed with us.

Living with cats, dogs, and snakes

Animals moved into Erika's home as well. It all began with a little tabby cat that the Superintendent's children found one day. They asked Erika if she'd like to keep it. Yes, she said, that would be lovely. Initially, sharing space in the nurses' quarters was a bit difficult, but then the two of them moved into Erika's new home. The cat, "Tigerli," was apt to cling to Erika, but soon began hanging around with male cats and promptly got pregnant. Still too immature, she had a miscarriage, but shortly afterwards Erika noticed that something was moving in Tigerli's belly again, so she prepared a nice safe place for her to give birth. Then, returning home one evening from the theatre in Lemana, Erika discovered a newborn tabby kitten on the cement floor of the terrace, and she named it "Nepomuk." He was a very special cat, not a cuddly animal at all, but very sensitive, and as alert as a watchdog. Erika recalled:

> Nepomuk appeared promptly when called, like a dog! When I called for him, he'd come running from the farthest end of the garden. One Sunday evening, I was listening to the radio and he was sleeping on a chair beside me, snoring like a machine. Suddenly, he jumped up and bounded out on to the terrace. I assumed it was a mouse, and opened the door. He looked at me, as if to say, "Are you stupid?" Then he ran around the terrace and along all the windows, until I turned on a light outside and had a look myself. At that moment, a man took off running from behind the house. Nepomuk had played the role of a watchdog!
>
> Another time, the behaviour of Nepomuk and his mother made me sure that something was wrong. I had just put out food for the two cats. Tigerli came very hesitantly and kept glancing at the fireplace, while Nepomuk froze and trembled, also fixing his gaze on the fireplace. I noticed a wet patch on his head and suspected that there was an animal in the chimney that had attacked him. A snake? I went and asked the neighbours to help. Armed with a gun and a club, we lit a fire in the fireplace and waited for the attacker, until finally a dead screech owl fell down from the chimney! From then on, Nepomuk reacted very nervously to every little sound. But he remained very affectionate. When my dear friend, the mother of the Medical Superintendent, passed away, I just sat there sorrowfully in my bed. Along came Nepomuk and licked my hand. Sadly, one morning he didn't come home, and he was missing from then on. Perhaps it was a snake…? He was six or seven years old.

Erika has a great fund of snake stories. When her house was built and her garden cleared, the snakes apparently failed to understand that this piece of bush land was now civilised country, and they remained in their ancestral territory. Whenever Nepomuk or Tigerli returned home

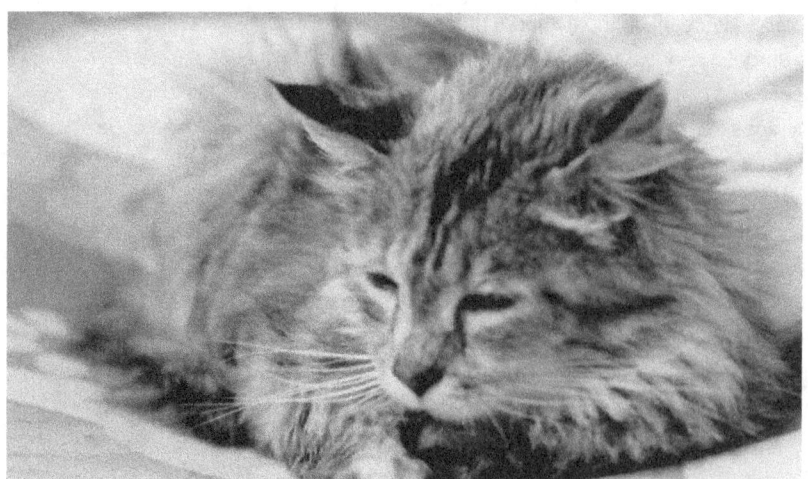

Erika's tabby cat, Nepomuk

with swollen eyes, it could only mean that they had run into a spitting cobra, or *rinkhals*, as they are also called. Luckily, they lived with an ophthalmologist, who put drops of milk in their eyes until they got better. Sometimes, in the early afternoon, a yellowish-grey cape cobra – two-and-a half metres long, and more poisonous than a black mamba – crawled around in the garden.

> Finally, Jackson discovered the hole that belonged to this snake. He poured in some petrol, threw in a burning match, and then dug and dug until he found the dead snake, rolled up in its den. That evening, another snake came along and searched the hole in desperation. We had never noticed they were a couple. From then on, the lone snake would always creep into the strawberry patch, and Hilda thought it was eating my strawberries. I disagreed, saying it was only eating the snails, which it was entitled to do. I had asked Jackson to hammer in some stakes around my two beds of strawberries and stretch nylon netting over them to protect them against birds. When I returned home, he proudly showed me what he'd created: a giant tent over the strawberries! If a bird happened to get through, Tigerli was lurking around ready to catch it. Then one day it happened that the cobra got caught in the nylon netting. Attempting to get free, it became more and more entangled until it finally strangled itself.

Later, in 1981, Erika also acquired a dog. One evening she and her brother Ernst, who was visiting her, came home to find the house in disarray. It has been broken into. The thieves were never found. Erika decided that it would be good to have a dog in the house as a deterrent. So a potbellied, brash little fellow named Mambuxu joined the household. He was a mixture of fox terrier and dachshund, with short legs and a head like a bull terrier. He endeared himself to Jackson, and eventually found a home with him in the village when Erika retired and returned to Switzerland.

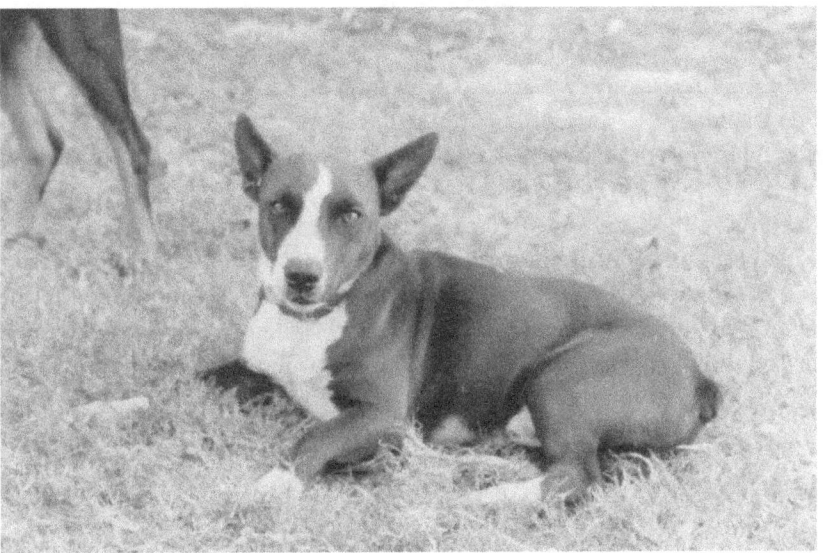

The dog Mambuxu

Guests at last!

Now that she had moved into her own home, Erika finally had the chance to welcome visitors and put them up, as well as to host parties, where usually everyone contributed something to the buffet. None of this had been possible before in the Nurses' Residence; it had always been necessary to find accommodation elsewhere for visitors. Now Erika could make good use of her memories of the Swedish hospitality that she had enjoyed so much during her time there as a researcher. There, it is common and natural to maintain an open home on account of the vast distances, and in South Africa it is the same. Erika's guests came with pleasure. They included her older brother Hans with his wife and daughter, and women friends from Switzerland, to whom she often entrusted her VW Beetle while she was at work in the hospital. On one occasion, she shocked her cousin on the very day she arrived, by offering two unknown men who were passing through a place to stay for the night. One of them introduced himself as physician, and said he had heard Erika give a lecture and wanted to get to know her. The two wanted to continue on over the border into Zimbabwe that evening, but Erika knew they couldn't make it in time before the border was closed. Without hesitation, she offered them dinner and prepared two guest beds – proceedings which her cousin observed wide-eyed.

Erika had to wait a long time for her younger brother Ernst to visit. He finally came in 1981, when she encouraged him to come for a Pan-African ornithology congress in Malawi. Erika was able to join the congress delegation from Johannesburg, and took advantage of the opportunity to observe innovative community health projects in Malawi. Afterwards, the two visited various game reserves in South Africa, and Ernst got to know Erika's work in Elim. He was so impressed by the country that he returned the next year with his wife Gaby. Since she enjoyed weaving tapestries, Erika planned a trip that became known in the family as the "weaver-bird-safari," during which they alternately visited game reserves and African weaving workshops. The two enjoyed themselves so much that they came back in 1984 for Erika's farewell celebration. Indeed, they wanted to know as much as they could about Erika's life in Africa and come to understand it better, in view of the future years when they would be together in Basel after Erika's retirement.

Making music in the mission setting

With her cello, her "baby," Erika took her love of music and active music making to Elim. Soon enough, a trio emerged among the mission workers, and they frequently put on small concerts there or in Lemana. Erika remembers an evening of baroque music in Lemana in which she clearly sensed how the African listeners were also moved by the music, though it was foreign to them. Her cello, "the great guitar," fascinated the Africans.

When Eveline Jacot, the skilled violinist from the trio in Elim, moved to a mission hospital called Masana, 300 kilometres to the east, Erika often drove there over the weekend to play in a quartet, and then returned home early on Monday morning. On the long, scarcely travelled road home, she kept herself awake at the wheel by singing. Indeed, singing worked magic, enabling Erika to win the hearts of the African nursing students. As soon as she sang a new melody with them, they sang it back to her in harmony. Their enthusiasm was contagious.

Vacation and more training

In 1969, four years after taking up her position as head ophthalmologist, Erika was able to take a year's leave for the first time. Capably serving in her place was a young Swiss ophthalmologist, Margrit Kellerhals, whom she had got to know while training in the Basel Eye Hospital. Among other things, Erika used the year for further training in Greenstead, England, to learn to carry out corneal grafts. The first patient that she could practise the surgical technique on in Elim was a ten-year-old girl who has been blinded by xerophthalmia. This form of blindness can occur within two days when a malnourished child with vitamin A deficiency gets measles. In such cases, the cornea softens and becomes gelatinous, and must be replaced with new tissue. To Erika's delight, the operation was a success and the child's sight was restored. In the following years, however, she very seldom performed this operation in Elim.

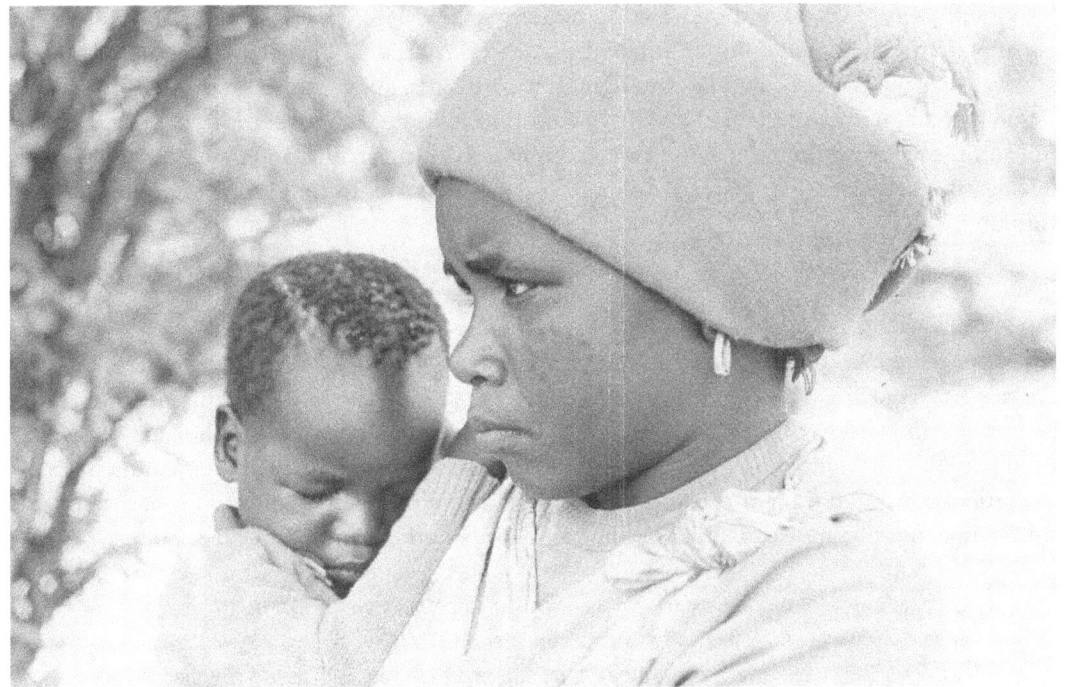

Measles in malnourished children with Vitamin A deficiency leads all too often to blindness due to xerophthalmia

Language – understanding – communication

Fortunately for Erika, when she returned from her leave in early 1970, Margrit Kellerhals was able to continue filling in for her for three more months, which finally enabled her to spend six weeks on an intensive study of Tsonga – a language that had become more and more important for her. She lived for a time in the nearby mission station Valdezia, enjoying language lessons from her old friend Irène Bourcart and from Rev. Theo Schneider, and conversation practice with a local teacher. Erika remembers:

> Theo Schneider had a particular gift for conveying the beauty of the Tsonga language and the manner of thinking that it expresses. In Tsonga sayings, the world often comes across as an animated, individual counterpart. One doesn't say, "I lost the path," but rather, "the path lost me." To orient oneself along a path, one doesn't speak of "a tree," but rather gives the name of the tree. One of our students jokingly referred to the consulting room in the hospital as the "snake park" – snakes are held responsible for many stomach ailments for which patients seek treatment. In the case of diarrhoea, for example, they are said to be "running around in the belly".

Observations of this kind reflect a set of beliefs that Europeans often wrongly interpret as superstition. Erika was fascinated by the ideas, but she ultimately remained aware that the foreign cultural mentality was only accessible up to a point, and her own language ability also had its limits. Though she learned a few standard phrases, it remained beyond her capacity to fully understand Tsonga and lead a conversation in it, and she still needed a translator for her work. Nevertheless, the Africans took great pleasure in Erika's ability to say simple things in their language. When she originally came to Elim in 1952, the hospital management attached no importance to promotion of indigenous language skills among hospital staff. In contrast, missionaries were required to study Tsonga intensively for six months as soon as they arrived. An additional problem was that patients came to Elim from three linguistic regions, speaking Tsonga, Venda, or Pedi (Northern Sotho). So where did one start? English, translated by African nurses, had to suffice. In 1972, the hospital management assigned translators to

Erika; Christina Tlakula and then the inimitable Selina Maphorogo. Later, as Erika's closest collaborator in the Care Groups, Selina intuitively translated only what she felt was appropriate and that the patients, and later people in the villages, appeared to be capable of accepting in a given moment. She had a real gift for building bridges between the medical personnel and the village women. Today, Erika comments, "It was a blessing that I couldn't speak Tsonga fluently, but that, instead, Selina translated things into the Tsonga people's way of thinking."

Explain, check, and explain again

Ever since she had completed her specialist training with Professor Rintelen in Basel, one of Erika's key concerns was to understand her patients and to be able to explain to them the symptoms and causes of their illness as well as the treatment strategies. She acknowledged each patient as a whole person and tried to involve him or her actively in the healing process, in particular through good information, discussions, monitoring of medication use, and follow-up. Things did not appear to be done the same way at other South African hospitals:

> I became aware of this, for example, when glaucoma patients were referred to me from Johannesburg. I would ask them what the doctor there had told them. The answer was always, "Nothing". They were given drops, they would say, and that was it. If I asked whether anyone had explained to them what they were suffering from, and why they needed to take the drops, I would receive the same answer, "No." It was always important to me that they understood why they had to take the drops for so long, so that they'd really do it – and would come back to be checked before their bottle of drops was completely empty. Otherwise they would stop, and go blind.

> Many of them didn't understand the need for long-term treatment of chronic diseases, so we had to emphasise repeatedly exactly what they needed to do. Once, I made rounds in the male ward and asked a glaucoma patient, "What will you do when you get home?" And I impressed upon him, once more, why he needed to take the drops regularly. Then the patient next to him wanted to know what he himself had. He had a cataract, so I told him that he had a different kind of disease that could only be treated by an operation, whereas the man in the neighbouring bed had a disease for which nothing could be done to improve his sight, but that he could still be prevented from going blind. And then it got going! All sixteen patients in the ward wanted to know which of the two diseases they had. They were all keenly interested, and we explained it to each of them.

> It wasn't the same with the women. They accepted their illness more fatalistically, and didn't ask about it. But I tried to explain things to them as well. One time, it was in 1970, I had a young woman with a unilateral cataract in front of me. In a young person, a unilateral cataract is usually the result of a trauma – for example, head injuries resulting from blows. I asked her if she had been beaten by her husband. She looked at me in astonishment. That was indeed what had happened to her. She was greatly impressed, because I had recognised that her husband had beaten her. So I played the role of the traditional healer, who often knows a lot about the patient's background.

A mischievous smile, maybe even the littlest bit proud, appeared at the corner of Erika's mouth, and grew as she related the following story:

> One morning, I came into the hospital while the patients were still eating breakfast. They sat in the hallway along the wall on their chairs, with their tin plates of maize porridge on their laps.

When I entered, one of the patients was putting on a little theatre show, because she was allowed to go home. She did a little mime to show how she had been when she came to the hospital, fumbling around blindly, and then performed a dance to show how vigorous she was now that she could see again and was going home. The other patients accompanied her, drumming loudly on their tin plates.

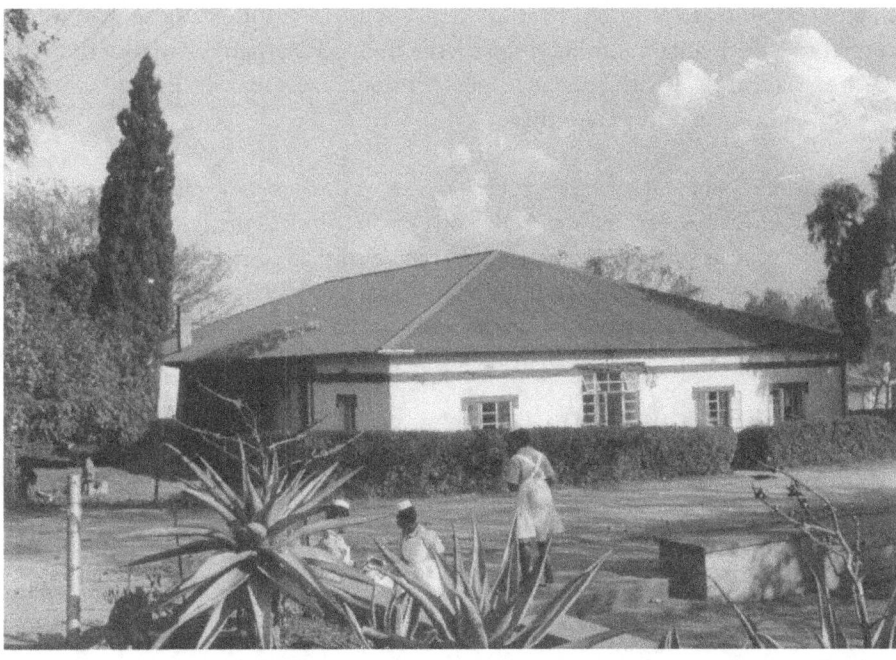

The Eye Hospital in Elim, 1968

In the same year, 1970, Ted Germond, Medical Superintendent at the mission hospital Morija in Lesotho, came to Elim to learn from Erika how to operate on cataracts. He was already an old friend, and she had spent holidays with his family in Lesotho. The collaboration was a pleasure and everyone liked him. When the two months were up, they gave a farewell party for him, at which he had to pass his "final exam":

> I constructed an eye out of an African drum about 50 cm high, using a piece of brown fabric for the iris. I draped it on so that it formed the circular muscle. A plastic bag stuffed with cotton wool served as the lens, which I put under the iris. At various points, I attached this "lens" so firmly that it was impossible to remove it from the eye without rupturing it. Ted was furnished with pliers and garden shears as surgical instruments, and given the task of extracting the lens.

Some time later, Dr Schmid came from Switzerland for a couple of months, giving Erika a chance to take another break. They also worked together for a time. She found it wonderful, for once not having to make every decision alone, and having the chance to discuss difficult cases with someone else. Their mutual learning was also useful. Dr Schmid, for example, needed to learn to adjust to the African conditions and not to lose his composure when medications were not promptly ordered, so that they were only available after a week or more had passed.

Stories about spectacles

Spectacles are highly regarded in the African context. For many Africans – just as for many Swiss people – they are seen as *the* remedy for all eye complaints, fatigue, or headaches. This is true in some cases, but often the problem has to do with patients' inability to focus both eyes on a point at close range. Normally, children automatically learn to focus between ages one and a half and two, using picture books and simple games. But this is seldom the case among the African children, since they are usually carried around on their mother's backs and their eyes don't receive the stimulation of picture books. As a result, lack of practice in focussing at close range is common in Africa, and this causes difficulties for children as soon as they enter High School and are required to study text books. In addition, those who wear glasses are perceived to be especially intelligent, a distinction which many naturally find attractive. So Erika often had to deal with spectacle prescriptions in Elim – or, indeed, with their absence. She tells stories that illustrate this:

> Many students from the nearby High School in Lemana came to us wanting glasses. When practice in focussing was all that was needed, I prescribed special exercises, which were often even fun. Most of the students were sceptical, of course, and I don't know if they performed the exercises long enough. However, one day, a student came with his girl-friend for a consultation, just to thank me. They hadn't believed me, they said, but the exercises had indeed helped, and now they could see well.

> On one occasion, a doctor from a neighbouring hospital referred a nine-year-old boy to me – a patient from his TB ward. According to the doctor, the boy's vision was getting worse and worse, but he couldn't find any cause for it. I examined the child and discovered that his vision was perfect. So what was the matter with him? I finally found out; another child on the ward had got a pair of glasses, and now he simply wanted a pair for himself.

> Sometimes, opticians were guilty of scams. Once, a nurse came to me in the clinic with the recommendation of her optician, who claimed she needed a new pair of glasses every year. When I measured her lenses, I discovered they were just plain glass! The name of the optician, a European, was printed in the spectacle case, and I was able to pursue the matter together with our Medical Superintendent, Pierre Jacques. He called the optician and asked him what the refraction was of the spectacles he'd prescribed, since he'd told his customer that she'd need new ones every year. Then the optician confessed that they were just plain glass. Her eyes were totally normal, but, "Blacks simply want to wear glasses to look intelligent". Of course, Pierre Jaques didn't tell the optician that we were calling from the eye clinic. Afterwards, I asked the nurse why she went to the optician, and whether she had wanted glasses. She claimed that that wasn't the case; she'd mainly gone to the optician because of frequent headaches.

Apartheid and forced resettlement

Since the late 1960s, the "resettlement" policies of apartheid have affected the lives of the African population, as the Black Sash and many other organisations in the protest movement pointed out critically from the very beginning. So what was it all about? The South African government's long-term goal at that time was to divide up the entire South African population by race, and the African population by ethnicity or language group. Land was allocated to each ethnic group, in areas called variously "Homelands" and "Bantustans". The apartheid government's aim was that the "Homelands" would become "fully independent" states. The impression that the people in Elim had was that the government wanted to abandon all responsibility for them. Eighty percent of the total population would be made to live on thirteen percent of South Africa's territory, while eighty-seven percent of the areas with the richest soil were in the possession of the European minority. The Africans living in the poor and overpopulated "homelands" would provide a reservoir of workers.

The apartheid laws made segregation more systematic. One of the intended measures was to eliminate scattered African settlements – so-called "black spots" – in European areas, forcing the inhabitants to resettle without receiving any compensation for their land. The consequences were especially devastating for those African ethnic groups that had settled in the "wrong" places or had been living in communities where the ethnicities were mixed. They were split up and relocated to their respective Bantustans. For example, Tsonga people living in a region reserved for Venda were forced to move out, and vice versa for Venda living in an area designated for the Tsonga.

That nearly always meant moving from a better area to a region where there were no opportunities for work. The government's promises – that everything would be better in the new location – were revealed as fantasy. Nevertheless, the Xhosa peoples of the Transkei and then the Ciskei accepted the offer of "independence." They were later followed by the Venda and the people of Bophuthatswana. The citizens of these four "homelands" received passports from the government and were forthwith designated as belonging to independent states, though these were never recognised as such by the international community.

In 1969, Gazankulu (the Tsonga "homeland") opted for partial autonomy under Chief Minister Hudson Ntsanwisi – previously moderator of the Tsonga Presbyterian church – but refused to become an independent state. As a "self-governing territory" Gazankulu was given its own ministries of health, education, finance, and social affairs, yet it remained financially dependent on Pretoria, which also continued to be responsible for military affairs. Since Gazankulu had rejected full autonomy, it received less money from Pretoria than the adjoining smaller Venda territory. In this way, the government tried to exert pressure on Gazankulu. The wider changes resulted in considerable administrative complications for the hospital in Elim. The Gazankulu health administration bore the responsibility for the African staff members, while the central government in Pretoria was still responsible for the European employees.

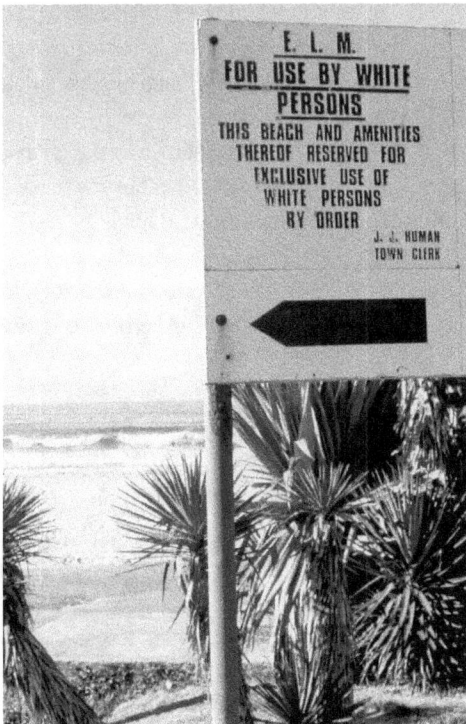

Racial segregation; sign on a beach in Durban, 1986

The resettlement actions in the Gazankulu region took place during the harsh winter of 1971. In some other areas, when a village community resisted resettlement, soldiers would show up with guns, threaten the residents, and bulldoze their homes to the ground. Fortunately, this did not happen in Gazankulu. The people were rounded up with their belongings and loaded into trucks for the trip to a new location in the east.

Erika recounted:

> Worst of all was the resettlement of the Makuleke people to Nthlaveni. They were relocated from the fertile territory along the Levubu River, north of the Kruger National Park, to a dry, uninhabited area west of the park that had been newly added to Gazankulu. There were also people from the villages around Elim who were taken there. From west to east, into country that became drier and drier. Rev. Jean-François Bill from Lemana travelled with them – a risky decision, as the government did not like anyone observing the resettlements. He later shared what he saw. The people were given nothing more than a few wooden poles and a bunch of grass with which to build a hut. They were simply unloaded in no man's land in the bitter cold. There were elderly people and children among them, and some of them died.

A Makuleke song[1] conveys the suffering experienced during resettlement:

> *Valungu va hi hlongola*
> *Valungu va hi hlongorile mayana kaya khoma ndlela*
> *Hi yowe ee hi ta sala na Makuleke ee khoma ndlela*
> *Hi yowe ee hina hi tele ku hela oo khoma ndlela*
> *Mi hi tekele ku ta hela oo mayana kaya khoma ndlela*
> *Hina hi tele ku hela mayana kaya khoma ndlela.*
>
> The Whites are chasing us away.
> The Whites have chased us away.
> We want to return home.
> We have come here with Makulele. We return home.
> Many of us have died. Take the road home.
> We have come here to be destroyed.
> We are all finished. Let us take the road home.
> You have taken us here to destroy us.
> We want to take the road home.[1]

An excerpt from Erika's newsletter of February 1971, about the resettlement to Nthlaveni, demonstrates the significance of the resettlement policy, in concrete terms, for people in the northern region of Elim:

> Nthlaveni is located about one hundred kilometres away from Elim, on the edge of the Kruger Park. The area receives little rainfall, even in normal years. Though it has good grassland, the soil is thin and not suitable for crops. The last ten years were dry, but the worst summer of all was last year, when there was no rainfall whatsoever. The people there live on maize, which they can buy if their men in the city send money home. During the drought, no wild vegetables grew, and the gardens could not thrive without water either. Malnutrition is so common that patients with milder symptoms are often described as "healthy".

The Presbyterian Church recognised the direness of the situation and began to set up soup kitchens for the poorest in the region, just as the Lutheran Church had done a bit earlier on behalf of the Venda. Erika's friend Irène Bourcart, from Valdezia, was given the task of organising the soup kitchens, and Erika was able to travel with her to Nthlaveni. She was not really allowed to enter the region without special permission, but she did so anyway, hoping to avoid being checked. The story of that journey still makes her very sad:

> Along the street lay bundles of "roofing grass" for constructing huts. An old woman had built herself a crude shelter out of grass, a sort of little igloo, for protection. Many children had pellagra, a sign of vitamin C deficiency. The conditions were miserable. We saw one small ray of hope; someone had already planted a touching little vegetable garden, fenced off with corrugated iron.

After they had distributed the soup, Erika went into the settlement with Irène. As soon as people heard that the "eye doctor" was there they began to come and talk to her. One of them was a former cataract patient from Elim. Just as she was about to examine him, a car pulled up – the dreaded magistrate! And there she was, without authorisation! There was nothing for the two women to do but introduce themselves:

> In Irène's case, there was no problem. For my own part, I simply said that I was the ophthalmologist from Elim, and that I was examining a former patient of mine. Then came the official's unexpected response: "Doctor, I want you to come here and see what is needed. Elim shall build a clinic here." A big sigh of relief! We did make an assessment in the area later. I went with the paediatrician, Dr Schibler, and our teams.

In the end, nothing came of the Elim clinic. The much nearer Tshilidzini Hospital, belonging to the Dutch Reformed Church, was given the contract to establish the out-station.

Apartheid and Christianity

Erika becomes very thoughtful whenever she recalls her memories of the resettlement activities. As a Christian, she is troubled to this day by the ugly truth that, from the very beginning, there were those who sought to justify apartheid by referring to the authority of the Bible. The Afrikaner Dutch Reformed Church – the *Nederduitse Gereformeerde Kerk* (NGK) – was also known as "the Nationalist Party at prayer", or the religious arm of the ruling nationalist party. It argued that apartheid was the Will of God. One theologian whom Erika greatly admires, C.F. Beyers Naudé, had grown up in this tradition, but nevertheless eventually chose a completely different path.

Encounters with C.F. Beyers Naudé

Erika encountered Rev. Beyers Naudé several times, and this gave rise to a special friendship that strongly influenced her attitude towards apartheid. She still has vivid memories of these encounters with "the Dom Helder Camara of South Africa", as she calls him, and his life story:

> Beyers grew up in a deeply religious, conservative Afrikaner family. His father held a high-level position in the Dutch Reformed Church and in 1918 was a co-founder of the *Broederbond*, a secret organisation that greatly influenced the seizure of power by the mainly Afrikaans-speaking Nationalist Party in 1948, and their enforcement of apartheid policies. For twenty-five years, Beyers was also a member of the *Broederbond*. He became a pastor, and was Moderator of the NGK for the whole of Transvaal. In the late 1950s, young European ministers from the NGK who were appointed to work in African or coloured congregations witnessed – for the

first time – the consequences of the apartheid laws. Troubled by what they saw, they brought their concerns to Beyers Naudé. Initially he was sceptical, but he did go to the communities to see for himself. What he found there shook him to the core, but he didn't dare to make any official statement. Then he began to study the Biblical texts that were used to justify apartheid and discovered that the texts – unconsciously or consciously? – had been bent to support the ideology of apartheid in such a way so as to make it appear absolutely plausible and correct for the church and its members. Yet Beyers still did not dare to make any official comment.

The turning point came in 1960. In March, an inter-confessional consultation of the World Council of Churches took place in Cottesloe, a neighbourhood in Johannesburg, at which decisive resolutions were passed regarding race relations. They were rejected by the delegates of the NGK, but some of their ministers, including Beyers, supported them. At the time, I was studying in Johannesburg and had the opportunity to attend some of the conference events. From then on, of course, I followed the further developments with keen interest. In December of the same year, 1960, the Sharpeville Massacre occurred, in which the police opened fire on a peaceful demonstration by Africans against the pass laws, killing sixty-nine people.

Beyers could no longer avoid taking a clear stance. In 1963, activist Christians of all denominations founded the Christian Institute, an organisation comprising many groups and individuals scattered across the country. I was a member of the Elim group. Beyers became the director of the Institute as well as the general secretary of the South African Council of Churches (SACC), which strongly opposed apartheid. Archbishop Tutu was a leading figure there. The Dutch Reformed Church (NGK) withdrew from the SACC and Beyers, still its Moderator, was expelled from the church. He was stripped of his cassock in front of his congregation – however, they continued to stand by him.

Erika with Ilse and C.F. Beyers Naudé on a visit to Jean-François and Molly Bill, 1986

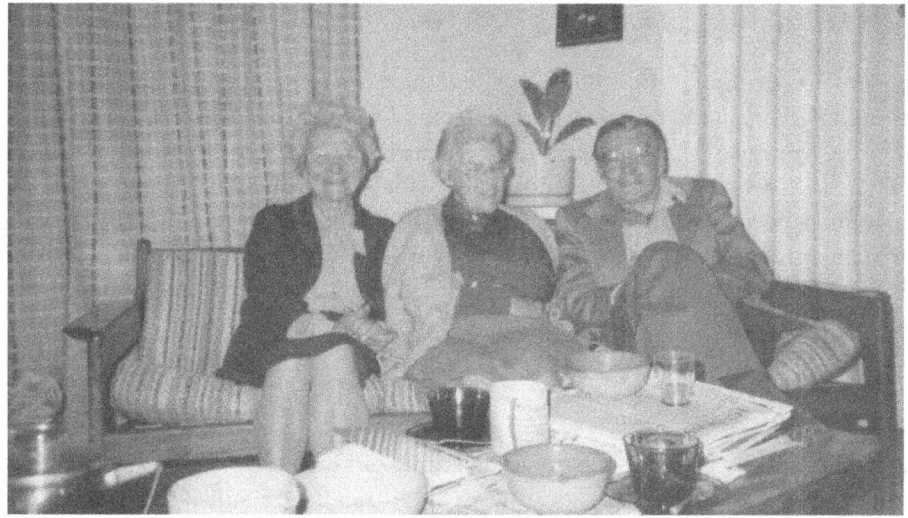

Around 1966, I became a delegate for the Elim Christian Institute group, and came into personal contact with Beyers in this way. We could occasionally invite him to the North for weekend lectures, sermons, and discussions. Once, he came to Elim for a week, and he and his wife Ilse stayed with me. Of course, spies were everywhere, and behind them the Secret Police. The day after the Naudés left Elim, the Secret Police turned up at the house of Rev. Mpfumu, the local pastor, asking for details about their visit, and where they had been staying.

Wherever Africans were subjected to police violence, Beyers would go, and he did everything he could to prevent such violence. The government watched Beyers, the Christian Institute, and the Council of Churches very closely, seeking an opportunity to accuse all three of them of inciting violence and attempting to overthrow the government.

The government did not succeed, however. In a lengthy trial in 1973, Beyers repeatedly emphasised that he could do nothing else. He had to obey God more than Man, or the State. Once, when I was leaving on vacation in 1974, Beyers gave me a thick envelope with instructions to send it to an address in Geneva. I was unaware that I was forwarding the secret records of proceedings at his trial to an international organisation of lawyers working for Human Rights.

In 1976, the Christian Institute was banned, and Beyers Naudé was served a banning order for an indeterminate time. This finally resulted in seven years of house arrest. The banning order specified the following: he could only speak with one person at a time, he was forbidden to set foot in institutions like universities or libraries, and he could not leave Johannesburg. He was stripped of his passport and had to report to the police every day. In addition, a dubious looking car often stood in front of his house for hours. It almost certainly belonged to the Secret Police. His telephone was tapped, and his home was very probably bugged. I witnessed all this myself when I visited him and his wife Ilse for a week once. Ilse had invited a German theologian to dinner, and when we sat down, Beyers said, "Don't be surprised if I pick up my plate and go and eat in the kitchen." He did that whenever he had a suspicion that someone was spying on them, since he was forbidden to speak with two guests at once. The other guest was speechless with astonishment! To maintain a little privacy, Beyers and Ilse usually kept all the shutters closed, and they left the radio on, to make it more difficult to monitor what they were saying through the bugs.

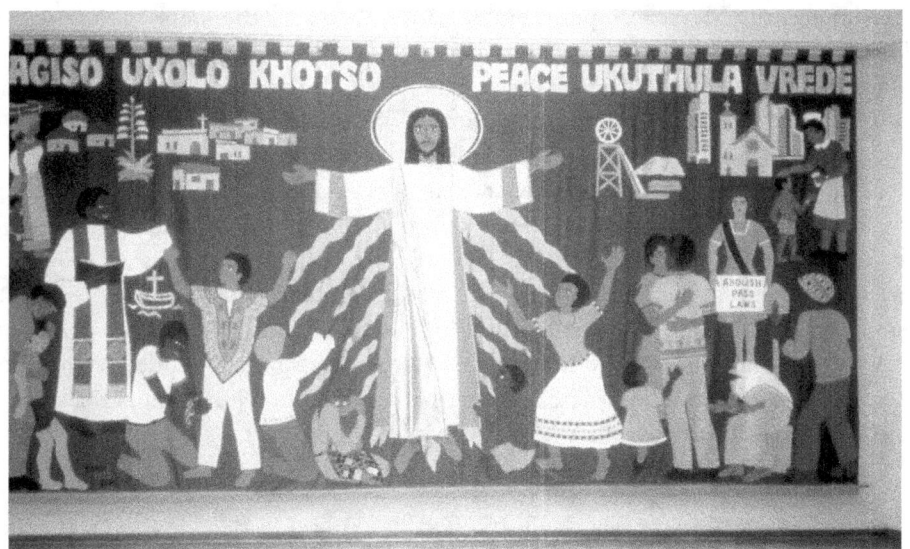

Peace wall-hanging in Khotso House, the headquarters of the SACC and the Black Sash, ca. 1982

In 1971, before the banning order, Beyers made an appearance at a Lutheran church about thirty kilometres from Elim, in the Venda area, and I drove there in the car with a few of the nurses. Along the way, the police were pulling over all drivers and asking them where they were going. I just lied and said we were on our way to a hospital in the area, and we were able to carry on without having our IDs checked. The discussions took place in the church. During the break we all went out for a breath of fresh air. I had to run back into the church to get something, and that was when I noticed Beyers on his knees, deep in prayer. It moved me deeply to see how he repeatedly gathered strength through prayer, and went before God on behalf of those suffering oppression.

Working and living in South Africa under apartheid

Nationalisation of the mission hospitals

Another of the apartheid government's systematic measures was to take over all mission hospitals. What began with nationalisation of the mission schools in 1952 was now being continued with the hospitals. Erika realised after reading a book on the powerful *Broederbond* – the driving force and "think tank" of the "white" government – that this was their recommendation. Many doctors at these hospitals – South African and foreign – were a thorn in their sides, because they often refused to toe the line and comply with apartheid policy. So the *Broederbond* urged the Government to take action against them.

In 1969, at the time when Erika was on home leave, Elim Hospital celebrated its seventieth anniversary, and a new hospital wing was opened. At the celebration, M.C. Botha, the Minister of Bantu Administration and Development, gave a speech in which he hinted at the planned nationalisation of mission hospitals. But it was not until 1973 that this actually occurred, and radical policies of racial segregation finally began to have profound effects on life at the hospital. There was a lot more bureaucracy, and thus higher costs, as a result of the new hospital organisation. Gradually, the relationship of trust between some of the European and African staff and patients also began to erode, and this sometimes resulted in a tense atmosphere, with both sides suspicious of the other. Where did the European doctors who were obliged to remain loyal to Pretoria really stand? And the mission? And the church? Erika asked herself these questions over and over, as did the rest of the staff.

Dr Pierre Jaques, the Medical Superintendent, formulated his thoughts on the matter in an essay for the staff. For him, the distinction between healing and curing was very important. To heal meant to restore the balance between body, mind, and spirit within the sick individual – in other words, to practise holistic medicine, which should be given the highest priority in a Christian hospital. In contrast, Western curative medicine, as practised in secular hospital settings, focussed solely on the body or on an organ – at best, perhaps a little on the mind – but ignored spirituality. In view of the government's unwavering intent to take over the mission hospitals, Dr Jaques suggested that it was the responsibility of the staff and the church to ensure that the spirit of healing remained visible. Erika shared this sentiment. Around 1969, medical missions worldwide had begun discussing the concept of a *healing community* that comprised the hospital and its entire environment. Elim had also made a brief attempt to go in this direction, but it quickly foundered. Nevertheless, the church maintained a strong presence in the hospital after nationalisation, just as it had before.

"I simply didn't let apartheid interfere with my work"

Erika has a special gift for simply getting on with her work, and she went on doing that in spite of the intensifying apartheid restrictions. She recounted several episodes to illustrate how difficult, sad, and sometimes ridiculous this could be:

> On one occasion, I had to operate on a European child, whose family were friends of the Liengme family. With the parents' permission, I did so in the hospital for Africans, where the operating room was better equipped and I felt more comfortable. Everything went well, but the Medical Superintendent, Dr Jaques, was not terribly pleased as it meant breaking the law.
>
> On another occasion, a doctor from Louis Trichardt asked me to look at one of his patients who had a very red eye. The doctor suspected glaucoma. I requested that the patient come to the

hospital that same afternoon, as a case of acute glaucoma should be treated immediately. I no longer had a consulting room for Europeans, so he had to come to the hospital for Africans, which was evidently something quite awful for him. When he arrived accompanied by his wife, I was in the middle of a conversation with an African social worker, and I asked the two of them to wait a moment. The conversation didn't last long, but I noticed how their faces grew redder and redder, especially when I shook hands with my African colleague as we said goodbye. Then, just as I began examining the patient, the electricity went out. Everything fell apart at that point. I did all I could for the moment, and told the patient that his case definitely wasn't an emergency and that he should kindly come again the next day, as I needed a slit lamp and electricity for further examination. But the couple had been so horrified by everything that of course they never returned.

As a result of apartheid, teaching and interacting with the African nursing students at the eye hospital gradually became more difficult. When I had to criticise them – just as I would have done at a Swiss nursing school – they immediately took it personally and thought to themselves, "She hates me because I'm an African."

When I returned to Elim as a doctor, I had more authority and it wasn't always easy for me to handle it comfortably. I was now in a senior position, running a more-or-less self-governing section of the hospital. There were times when I may have acted aggressively, especially when I felt unsure of myself.

In the period around 1979–80, Venda was on its way to becoming a Bantustan, an "independent" National State. It was very loyal to Pretoria and was favoured by the apartheid government, which gave it preferential treatment when allocating resources – in contrast to Gazankulu, which received less because it did not want to become fully independent.

Erika recollects:

Shortly before the vote, the head of the Venda government, Mphephu, had all of the key opposition members arrested to prevent them from voting or being elected. But there was not enough space in the prisons, so many of these opposition members – most of them teachers – were held captive in schools under terribly unhygienic conditions. While I was away on vacation, some of these prisoners came to the hospital with red eyes, and our nurses admitted them, even though it was not really necessary. They knew, of course, that I would have agreed to take them in, and that's what I continued to do when I got back. Soon word got out among the political prisoners that one need only rub one's eyes vigorously, until they turned red, to get out of prison and go to the Eye Hospital. So I practised a bit of sabotage!

Erika also experienced the mounting pressure of apartheid in her private life. She recalls several examples:

Every year, I had to report to the government office in Louis Trichardt in order to renew my driver's licence. The office had a small partitioning wall meant to separate Europeans from Africans. On my side, a woman employee took care of the various formalities in a fast and friendly manner. Beside me, an African man was making the same sort of request as I was, but he barely had a chance to open his mouth before the woman snarled at him. I held my tongue.

However, on another occasion I did show more courage. I had to go to my bank on the last Saturday of the month, a day I usually avoided, because it was when everyone got their paycheques from their employers, and had to go to the bank to cash them. Barclay's Bank didn't have an official policy of separating Africans and Europeans at the counters, but it happened anyway. I was standing in the middle of a long queue of Africans, when the cashier gave me a sign that I should proceed to the rear counter. I didn't react. A bit later another bank employee came over to me personally and asked me to go to the other counter so that I could be quickly served. I replied loudly, for all to hear, "I don't jump the queue because I am European." You should have seen people's reactions! The Europeans went about their business with angry expressions, and the Africans all beamed and laughed.

Could Erika be viewed as being subversive? The examples seem to suggest it, but she herself has this to say:

You can't portray me as being so brave! When we were growing up, I let my sister fight on my behalf against parental decisions that seemed unjust. I only gradually learned to fight, later in life. In part, I was just too timid to state my position openly. As an example; Pierre Jaques once said that he never knew quite what I was really thinking. It was a weakness of mine that what I said was often ambivalent, and I was nervous about speaking out. Once, however, I felt very comforted about my weakness. At a meeting between Elim's Christian Institute group and Beyers Naudé, one of the people attending told him that she could never be as brave as he was. His response was, "Not everyone must be; it isn't in everyone's nature." Nevertheless, the Africans knew and could feel where I stood. I simply did what was necessary at each moment and didn't pay any attention to the apartheid rules that were encroaching on every part of life.

New possibilities open up: a second ophthalmologist in Elim

In 1972, at the request of Dr Jaques, the government approved and agreed to finance a post for a second ophthalmologist at Elim hospital. This eventually gave Erika more time to broaden the scope of her work. A partnership began to emerge with the Basel University Eye Hospital in 1974. Following Professor Rintelen's retirement as Head of the Basel Eye Hospital, his successor, Professor B. Gloor, succeeded in gaining accreditation from the Swiss Medical Association (FMH) for a year of specialised training under Erika in Elim. This made a year

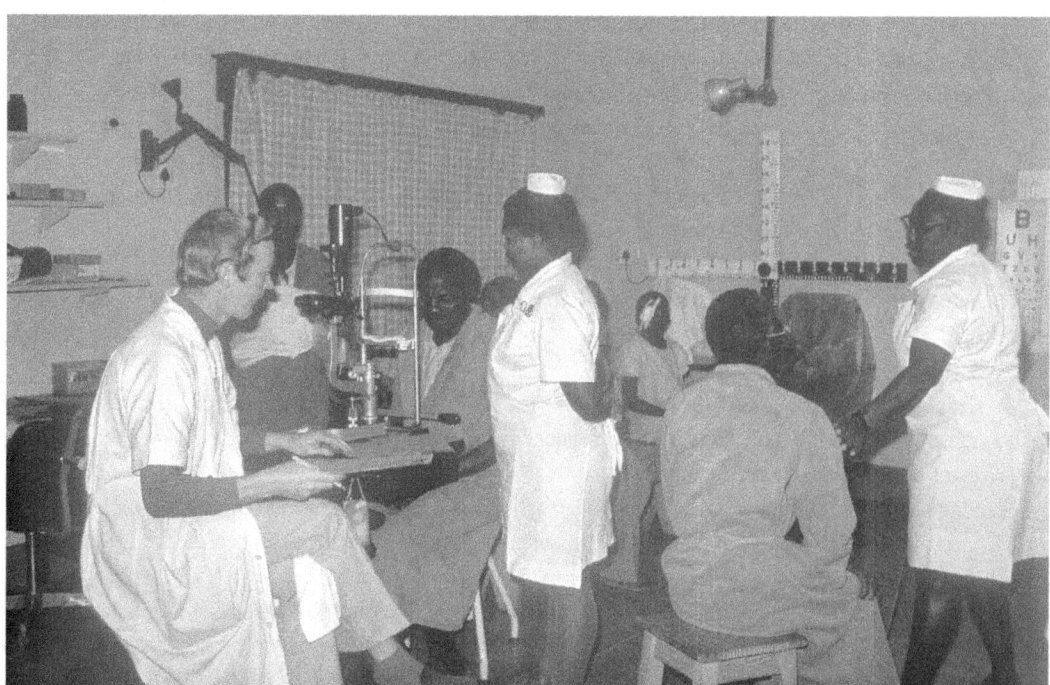

The second Opthalmologist in Elim, Dr. F. Käppeli, at the slit lamp, assisted by Christina Tlakula, 1974

of service in Elim more attractive, since it counted towards the clinical experience required for a specialist qualification in ophthalmology. Doctors in their last year before qualifying started coming in almost uninterrupted succession, most of them staying from one and a half to two years.

The first to come were a husband and wife, Franz and Ute Käppeli, both ophthalmologists. A particular achievement of theirs was the introduction of monthly eye consultations at four other hospitals in the region, done by one of Elim's ophthalmologists on a rotating basis. They were followed by Hansjörg Michel-Walser, his wife Ursina, and their two children. When Erika saw Ursina, she recognised her immediately – she was the daughter of Rev. Walser, a pastor in Davos, and Erika had met her as a four year-old when she was working at the meteorological observatory there when she was a student. Ursina still had the same head of curly blonde hair, and big blue eyes.

Having the assistance of a second doctor was a huge relief. Erika appreciated being able to discuss things with a colleague and sharing the responsibility. And it was very reassuring for her to know that somebody else could do the more complicated operations, because soon after the second ophthalmologist arrived, Erika began to have problems with her own eyesight. Now that eye consultations were available in four more hospitals many more patients could be reached, and surgery was performed almost every day, instead of only on two days per week. The number of cataract operations almost quadrupled, and, thanks to a surgical microscope donated from Bern, Switzerland, more glaucoma patients could also be treated surgically.

The other important result of having competent medical colleagues was that at last Erika was able to start turning three long-held dreams into reality: the training school for a diploma in ophthalmic nursing, the Rivoni rehabilitation center for the blind, and the establishment of community health work – starting with eye care – in the surrounding villages. Up to this point, she had had no spare time to implement her ideas, or to take a longer leave, because there was nobody else to do the work.

The School for the Diploma in Ophthalmic Nursing

This was the first of the three projects to be realised. It was something Erika had dreamed of for a long time – indeed, the idea had been in the back of her mind since her first working day as an ophthalmologist in Elim, when she had happened to overhear a Nursing Council inspector ask the matron, "Why don't you have a nursing school for eye care here, too?" Elim Hospital had had a nursing school for Africans ever since 1933, providing exceptionally good training – even compared to Swiss standards at the time. The school had official accreditation from the South African National Nursing Council. The addition of a training school for ophthalmic nurses had to remain a dream for eight years, due to the demands of existing work. But in 1975 a door opened at last. Erika could implement her plan and open a nursing school for eye care within her department.

On March 1st 1975, the South African Nursing Council granted their authorisation. At the school, qualified nurses would be eligible to complete an additional one-year training program in eye care and finish with a diploma. Despite the high demand, only three students were admitted at the beginning of the first course cycle, followed by three more students for the second cycle, launched six months later. For the hospital's ophthalmologists, planning and teaching lessons at the school meant a completely new, additional set of tasks. Management of the school and the lion's share of the teaching were taken on by Sister Tutor Tsakani Baloyi, who handled the work with great aplomb.

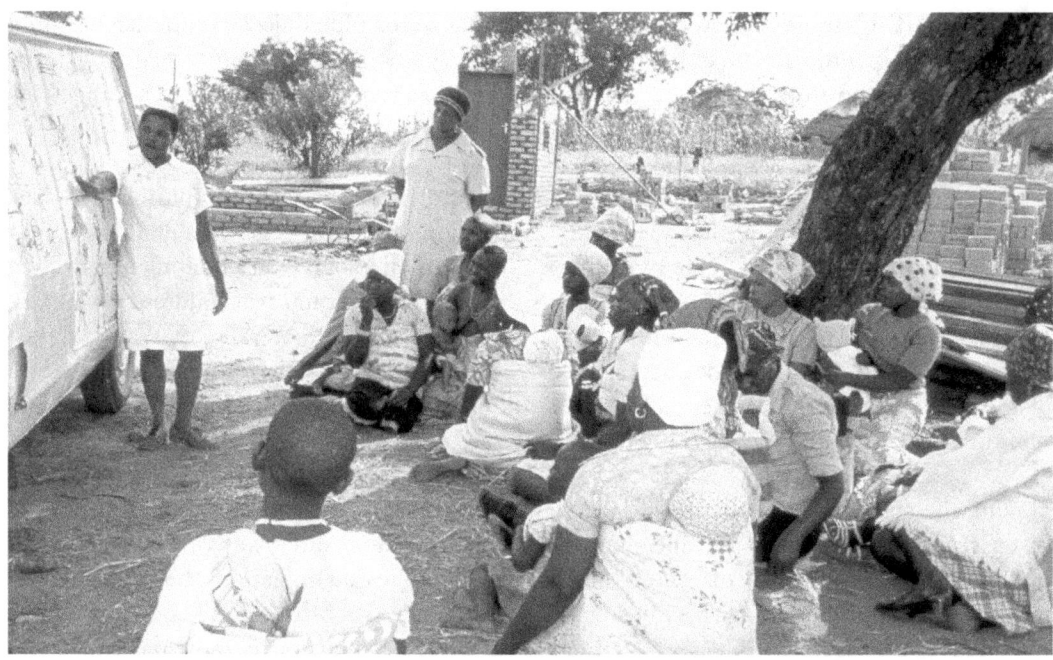

Health education for patients waiting in front of a clinic. Nursing Assistant Christina Tlakula is talking about trachoma, the main cause of avoidable blindness in the area, 1974

The founding of the school gave Erika the opportunity to design a course of study that would give due credit to the competence of the African nurses. In years past, she had repeatedly found African nurses trained in Elim to be very well qualified compared to their European counterparts, and often even better, and she had seen their outstanding nursing and organisational skills as well as their ability to observe accurately and react quickly. She trusted them, and encouraged them gradually to assume more responsibility. Often enough in her work in the hospital she had witnessed difficult and even grotesque situations that arose when skilled African nurses had to work under less competent European ones, who, being "whites", were automatically given senior positions upon arrival. Erika was determined that the ophthalmic nurses should be able to take initiatives and exercise responsibility, and she therefore introduced two important additions to the curriculum:

- The theory and practice of Community Eye Care was included as a compulsory subject. Later on, this enabled the eye nurses to participate in the health-care work of the Care Groups.

- Qualified ophthalmic nurses should no longer merely assist the doctors, but should be allowed to diagnose and treat common eye ailments.

This new curriculum was officially recognised by the South African Nursing Council. Reflecting on it later, Erika concluded:

> Everyone truly benefited. For example, the ophthalmic nurses examined the patients on arrival, treated common ailments and did entropion repairs. In the end, they became better at the frequent trachoma-related eyelid surgery than the doctors, because it was a routine for them. When they graduated, I personally presented each of them with a special certificate expressing my satisfaction with their ability to do this or that.

> When they returned to the hospitals which had sent them for training, most of the nurses did have a chance to use their new skills. At one hospital, the ophthalmic nurse was even provided with her own consulting room, and a few beds in the wards were set aside for eye patients.

There was only one place where the doctors did not allow nurses to examine and treat patients, with the result that people needing immediate specialist attention for problems like laceration of the cornea were referred to Elim much too late, when their eyesight could no longer be restored. This was a tragic case of "doctor's superiority complex". Our trained nurses knew which patients had to be brought to an eye hospital immediately.

With the growing volume of work resulting from the nursing school and other projects, being able to delegate became increasingly important to Erika. The necessity was highlighted when Elim was without a second ophthalmologist for about a year. She recalled:

> When the last colleague left, he recommended that I simply give up the nursing school for the time when I would be alone. "That's the last thing I'll do!" I answered, as I was worried that it might be difficult to find another ophthalmologist after my retirement. And what would happen to our patients then? So once I was the sole remaining doctor, I had no alternative but to entrust even more of the work to the nurses. It needed a good deal of courage, and above all trust in the nurses' abilities, to delegate jobs to them that used to be done only by a doctor, in spite of the risk that mistakes might be made.

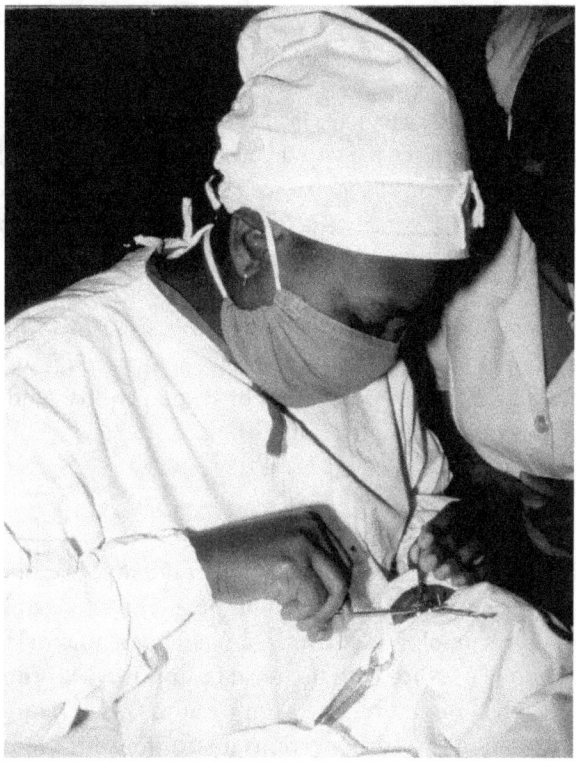

Nurse Vicky, the first student of the School for the Diploma in ophthalmic nursing, performing an entropion operation

> One demanding activity that I delegated was the running of the monthly consultations in other hospitals. I informed all the hospitals concerned by telephone that I was alone, and suggested that to bridge the time until a new doctor arrived I would send them my best students to perform the monthly consultations. All the Superintendents agreed. I talked to all the ophthalmic nurses and explained to them what they would have to do. At first, they were somewhat unsure of their ability to conduct the monthly consultations. "Of course you can do it!" I assured them. One evening when one of them, Nurse Minah, reported back after her day at Donald Fraser Hospital I asked her, "How did it go? What do the patients say when no doctor comes?" She answered quite spontaneously, "Oh, they like it much more when I come!" The reasons were

obvious. It was a Venda hospital where, because of the language, I was incapable of communicating with the patients without a translator, and the nurses could speak directly to them, which, of course, was much nicer. And the nurses had more time – when I was there, in my rush to get through about a hundred patients a day, it was always a case of "next, next, next" because of all the spectacles I had to prescribe, which the nurses weren't required to do. Africans are particularly good at languages, and the nurses could speak Venda, Tsonga, and Sotho fluently. My trust in them gave them self-confidence, and the monthly consultations in the four hospitals ran smoothly.

I always kept the Nursing Council informed about what I was doing, and they assured me that they approved, and that I was acting according to their regulations, which said that nurses could legally carry out all treatments for which they had been trained, and they could decide for themselves whether they were ready to perform a particular treatment.

However, my colleagues in the South Africa Council for the Blind (SACB) in Johannesburg were very sceptical about nurses performing operations. So, some years later, when I was due to go on leave for three months, and I was still the only ophthalmologist, I appealed to the Council to send one of their doctors to Elim for a day every two to three weeks to attend to problem cases, as long as the Eye Hospital was being run entirely by the nurses. But did any of my colleagues appear? No, not one of them!

When I returned after three months, I found that my confidence in the nurses had been fully justified. They made rounds with me, introduced me to all of the patients, and reported what they had done with them. They certainly hadn't made many more mistakes than I might have made myself! They had done really well, and were justly proud of what they'd accomplished. They had kept the tough cases for me, of course.

Erika beamed with pride as she related this story! And she has every right to be proud of her unwavering pioneering work in training, acknowledging, and gaining recognition for her African nursing staff. Her delegation of responsibility paid off – now six times more patients could be reached than before.

The Rivoni Society for the Blind

In 1975, Erika also fulfilled another of her dreams: establishing a much-needed rehabilitation center for visually impaired and blind people in the vicinity of Elim. In 1974, once there was a second ophthalmologist at Elim, she had been able to start planning the Rivoni Workshops for the Blind. Together with the local pastor, Rev. Mpfumu, she had preliminary discussions with the Elim community. She then went to Switzerland on leave for a year, and was able to gather inspiration by visiting various institutions for the blind. By the time Erika returned to Elim, Rev. Mpfumu had made good progress. He had set up an ecumenical planning committee, with mostly African members. This became the Rivoni Society for the Blind, an umbrella-organisation for a variety of activities. Before they laid the foundation stone, the committee members went on a joint trip to visit Transvaal's only workshop for the blind, which was near Pretoria. About three hundred blind people were employed there, and another three hundred were on a waiting list. The director of the workshop, blind himself, was more than happy to supply the group with helpful suggestions.

In 1975, Rivoni was ready to open its doors. From the beginning, it featured a carpenter's workshop which made coffins which were much in demand. People were pleased to be able to purchase a good looking coffin for very little money – much less than they would have had to pay an undertaker. In addition, the workshop produced beautiful candles, sisal doormats, and imitation-leather Bible covers, all of which generated a modest profit. The project also established a chicken farm, and acquired a nearby piece of land where blind people could cultivate vegetables for sale. A bit further away, in Venda, two large scale agricultural projects were set up, primarily for growing peanuts. Families, mostly headed by a father who was blind, were resettled here, where they could make a modest living.

It was no accident that Rivoni was opened near Elim Hospital – that made it possible for hospital patients who were incurably blind to be given guidance in managing household tasks, and "tips and tricks" for coping with everyday life. At Erika's request, such courses were later offered to patients of the Eye Hospital as well.

Sadly, the auspicious start to the Rivoni workshop for the blind was overshadowed by one big problem:

> I was a member of the Management Committee of Rivoni. We appointed an expatriate technician to manage the workshop. Some of us knew him, but we were not aware that he could be very violent. At first he did the job well, and he assumed responsibility for supervising construction besides introducing the first projects. But then I began receiving more and more complaints that he was prone to angry outbursts, and would hit people. It was really bad. I talked to him, and tried in vain to persuade the committee to act. It became clear that the situation was untenable and that he had to be dismissed. He then found another job, far away from Elim.

Following a long vacancy, shortly before Erika's retirement, a very competent European couple took over the management. They finally transferred the job to African hands several years later. A much wider range of activities was introduced, including Mobility Training, using a special long cane designed for use on uneven ground in rural areas.

A school was also founded, by Samuel Hlungwane, a former evangelist who was blinded by measles as a child and was one of the first five patients recruited from the hospital. There was a primary school for blind children in the area, in Siloe, but it only took children under eight years old. The Rivoni school took in children whose blindness began – or was diagnosed – when they were older. An agreement was reached with schools in the region that they would integrate the children into the normal school system once they had received enough special support. While at Rivoni, the children mainly learned to read Braille, and how to use a typewriter, which they were allowed to keep when they left to go to a normal school. One aim was to prevent the children from being isolated as disabled people, and instead enable them to live with their families and feel like normal people. At the same time, the sighted people around them were encouraged to get over their sense of unease and realise how much blind people are capable of.

There were also young people who came back to Rivoni because they had reached school-leaving age, but wanted to continue their education. They worked in small classes of about ten, and some of them even passed the Matriculation examination, which qualifies pupils for university entrance.

The positive development of the Rivoni projects has continued far beyond Erika's retirement, up to the present day. Visiting in 1995, she was amazed by how things had developed:

> About a thousand people have already completed the Mobility Training, and they come together each year for a rally in Elim, which includes a race! Over the years, Rivoni has developed

a new emphasis in its education of the blind and visually impaired. People are invited to come to the workshop for short-term training courses, typically for three months, offered by the Rivoni Society for the Blind. During this period, they learn Braille, management skills, and a trade. Ideally, they learn to do something practical that they can continue at home – for example, manufacturing the wire coat-hangers needed by dry cleaners in Louis Trichardt.

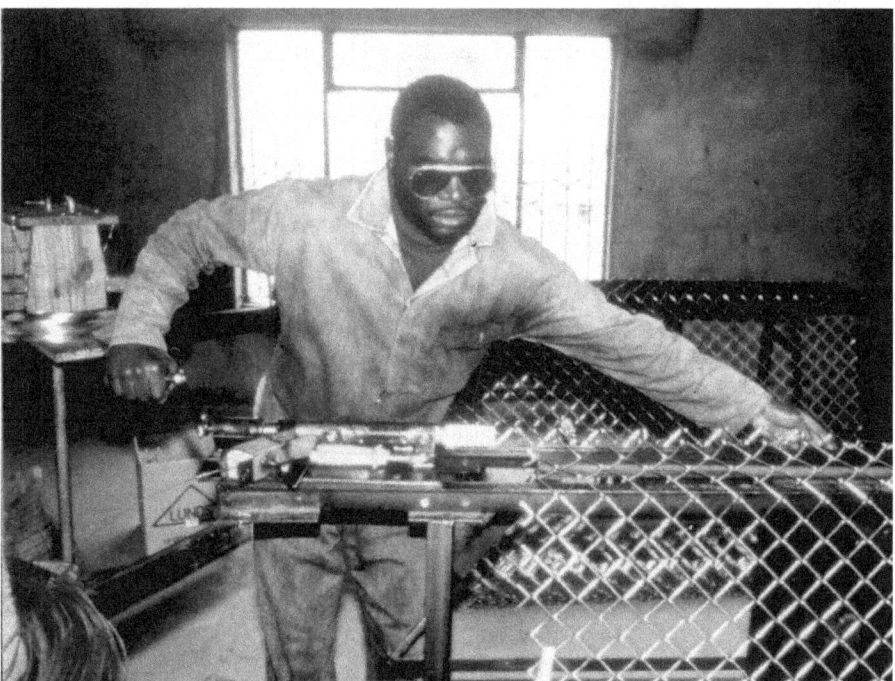

One of the village-based units producing metal fencing, run by a group of visually-impaired people

One of the most important activities of workshop participants is learning to make diamond-mesh wire fencing to protect gardens – a key commodity. There are now workshops for the manufacture of these fences in several villages, which are going very well. Five or six blind or visually impaired people set up a workers' co-operative, and Rivoni furnishes them with a wire-braiding machine and a supply of wire to start with, and also provides them with guidance and advice regarding management. After three months, the group must continue on its own, having established a basic means of earning a livelihood. I visited two such workshops and was very impressed. And the workshops provide a service for the people in the village, too, because they are able to buy fencing material more simply and cheaply than they could in neighbouring towns, and without paying a lot for transport.

The latest project started in 2005; Rivoni now has a bakery whose bread is in high demand throughout the area. So the Rivoni project's initial difficulties have gradually given way to what is now a true success story.

Preventive work; taking Eye Care into the community

It was only when her workload within the hospital was reduced at last that Erika finally had more time to invest in preventive medical work, which had become a pressing concern. Her original focus was on the control and prevention of trachoma, which was widespread in the region and was the most important cause of preventable blindness. Trachoma is a disease that arises out of poverty, lack of knowledge, and poor hygienic conditions. Curative medicine cannot eliminate the causes. This cannot be done without involving the affected population and getting their cooperation.

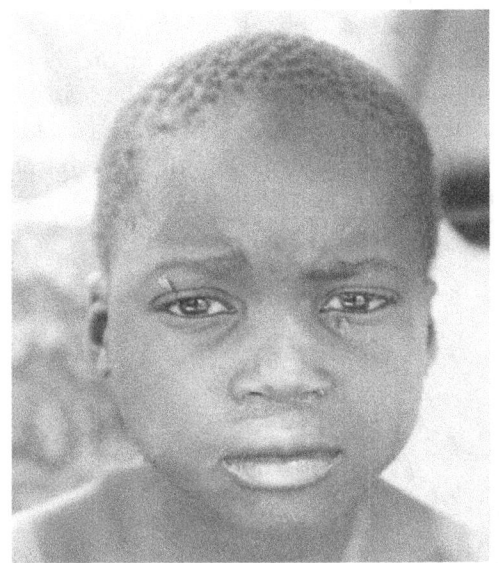
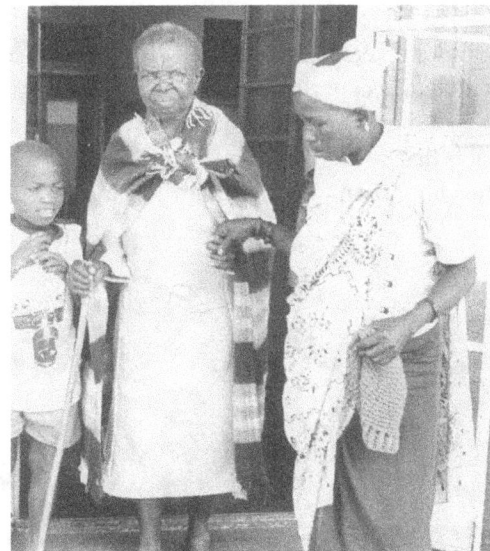

Left:
Early stage of trachoma. The ocular discharge attracts flies

Right:
Blindness in late-stage trachoma

Looking back, Erika said:

> For many years at the Eye Hospital I did my best to practice good curative medicine, as was the norm in mission hospitals in my day. My records of the patients coming for consultation revealed a high incidence of trachoma – but this was only the tip of the iceberg, as I later discovered through population surveys. Only two percent of the affected population came to the hospital, and I was almost exclusively dealing with the late effects of this chronic disease. People often accepted the disease as something that they just had to live with. Their eyes burned, and they rubbed them, but they didn't complain much until their eyelids began to fold inward, causing the eyelashes to rub on the eye. This is referred to as entropion, and eventually leads to blindness. Only when the condition was already bad did they come to the hospital. So I realised that it was necessary to come out of the hospital and go to the people – there, where the disease starts – in order to reach those who could still do something to prevent it.

This insight marked Erika's decisive turn along the path towards community health. Were there already approaches and experiences in this direction to draw upon? Two of her Dutch colleagues at Elim Hospital, Peter Kok and Rien Verhage, provided inspiration. They had already received training in primary health care while studying in the University of Groningen, in the Netherlands. In the medical school there, people had begun to realise that Western, curative medicine was not enough and that another approach was needed, one that worked with the people at a more fundamental level. Erika and her two Dutch colleagues formed a team that sought to blaze new trails. They also drew lessons from the sole contemporary book on primary health care, which became their "Bible": Maurice King's book on *Medical Care in Developing Countries*.

The South African Council for the Blind in Johannesburg already had some experience with trachoma. Under the direction of Dr G. Scott, a leading authority on the subject, field studies were conducted on the prevalence of trachoma as far back as 1955 in the region of Sekhukhuniland, revealing it to be a major problem in South Africa. From then on, broadly-based examinations of school children had been carried out widely, and treatment with tetracycline ointment was administered by teachers in the classroom. This did indeed reduce the infection, but children just beginning school were continually showing up as new cases. Why was this? Ron Ballard, a virologist at the Medical Research Institute in Johannesburg, provided a decisive answer. He had been appointed by the state to conduct a study on precisely that issue. He found that while the disease was declining among school-age children, preschool children were being infected with trachoma at home. Unfortunately, the Council for the Blind failed to accept the implications of the study, and continued with their projects in the schools. Erika found herself in disagreement with the Council, because she had come to the conclusion that it was important to reach children before they started school – and the best way of reaching them was through their mothers. So she took the next crucial step.

Transmission of trachoma through flies in pictures and in reality

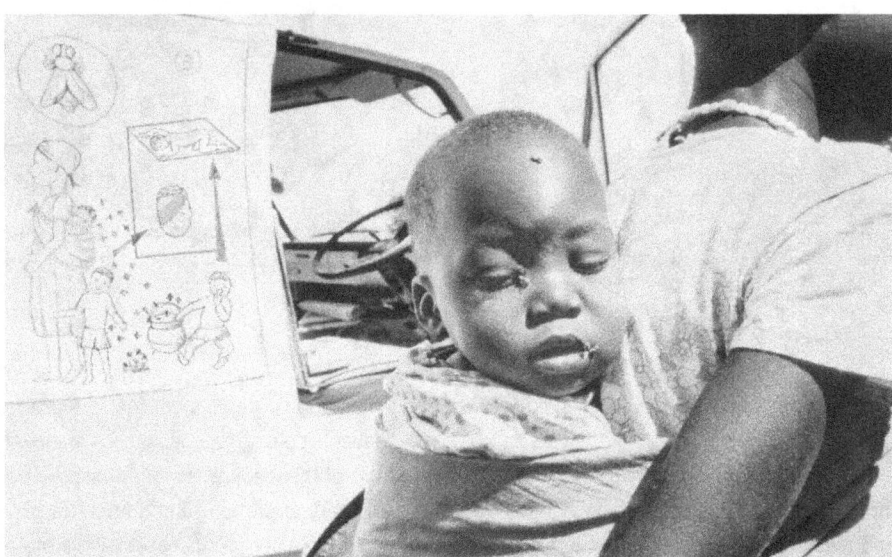

> There were some under-fives clinics to advise mothers, but these did not yet cover the whole area, which meant that not all infants and small children were included. So the idea arose of doing something in the villages. I had once read an article from North Africa about the training of health educators. They were taught that they should visit families in the evenings, when they were sitting around the fire, and talk to them about health problems like trachoma, and how diseases could be treated. I thought we could put something similar together ourselves, and came up with the idea of the Care Groups. We wanted to reach the mothers.

Erika began village work together with Peter Kok. He had already gathered experience, conducting a regional study of malnutrition, and now he joined Erika in her studies of trachoma. They did the work in their spare time, together with a few volunteers, as the Medical Superintendent, Dr Jaques, initially did not endorse the community health care approach – and a lot of their colleagues thought they were just taking walks in the countryside and leaving others to do the work in the hospital. Dr Jaques soon changed his view, however, and gave his full support to community health care. The way this project developed is described in detail in Chapter 7.

The Eye Doctor's own eye problems

These years of expanding work, when she could at last share the responsibility for the hospital and start on new projects, were very fulfilling ones for Erika. However, they were overshadowed by concerns about her own eye health. The first shock was in 1975:

> We were driving to the Donald Fraser Hospital, where we held a monthly consultation. I suddenly noticed that something was different. I could see the landscape just as before, but it had changed somehow. While I was measuring the patients' visual acuity at the hospital, I measured

> my own, and found that with my left eye I could just make out the biggest letters. It scared me, of course! Back at home that evening, I asked my colleague Franz Käppeli to look at my eye. The cornea was fine, but then he said with concern: "Why, there's a hole in the macula!" I was able to phone Professor Luntz in Johannesburg that same evening, and he recommended that I come to him at the hospital immediately. When I got there, everything was ready. The first examination revealed that I had a very rare form of macular degeneration. At that time, nothing could be done about it. A small cyst forms over the yellow spot, or macula lutea (the area of the retina with the largest concentration of photoreceptor cells), and as long as it remains intact, you continue to see well. But when it bursts, it leaves behind a hole in the macula lutea. I had to stay five more days in the hospital to undergo further examinations. They tried to comfort me by saying that it practically never occurred in both eyes. But that was precisely what happened, five years later. Ophthalmologists do come down with the rarest eye diseases!

For the moment, Erika could still see perfectly with her right eye, and when she returned to Elim she was able to continue working almost normally. But five years later, in 1980, she had another shock; her right eye suddenly began to give trouble. She knew she must consult a specialist at once, but it was the Thursday before Easter – and the next day was Good Friday, and a public holiday. However, when she telephoned Dr Kriel, the ophthalmologist in Pietersburg, he said he could receive her at the hospital for a consultation:

> I had already made plans for the day. The funeral for the father of one of my nurses was going to take place in a small village halfway between Elim and Pietersburg, 140 kilometres away, and I had promised to take the nurses who wanted to attend in my car. We drove to the village as planned, but instead of going to the service I apologised to the bereaved family, explaining that I would have to continue on my way to the doctor, and drove on. Then misery befell me. I was alone! The road's median strip looked like a zigzag line, and I knew then that I would never see a straight line again. Once at the hospital, Dr Kriel examined me. It was precisely the same diagnosis as with my left eye, even though this problem had hardly ever been known to occur in both eyes.

> I gradually had to accept that I couldn't be the same ophthalmologist as before. Using the microscope, I could just manage to perform cataract surgery. This was a routine operation. But I restricted myself to simpler procedures, and left the rest to my residents. They were very pleased to be able to perform more operations. At first, I operated together with them, and then later I left it to them, with sporadic supervision. I also had great confidence in the ophthalmic nurses, who were doing a lot of the routine work in the hospital.

For Erika, the emphasis of her work was already less on the curative activities within the hospital than on the outreach work in her various projects. Delegating work within the hospital enabled her to spend more time outside it. It was important for her to be mobile, though, and she was glad that she was still able to drive until her retirement in 1984. However, she did say that:

> On longer trips, I was always accompanied by a "co-pilot," one of the Care Group motivators, who alerted me to difficult situations.

Endnote

1 Patrick Harries: *A forgotten corner of the Transvaal: Reconstructing the history of a relocated community through oral testimony and song.* Presented at the University of Witwatersrand History Department in Johannesburg, February 1984.

VII The most meaningful years in Erika's life: The Care Groups

Chapter contributed by Frances Lund

Community eye health – the development of the Care Groups

Erika values the last eight years in Africa, during which the idea of community eye health through the Care Groups was developed, as the most worthwhile ones in her life. She reflects:

> It was the part of the work that made the most sense, for me and for the others, even when I thought I was doing it all wrong. While I was there I did not realise how much it was a development for me as well. When I started with eyes in Elim, like everyone I had a purely curative approach. The community approach was a great enrichment for me personally.

Ironically, the quarrel with the Council for the Blind over their school treatment method prompted Erika to try something better. The survey on trachoma in the Bungeni area provided her with the scientific foundation and authority to go ahead with a new method, based on the epidemiological pattern of trachoma in her area. As the young pre-school children are the ones who spread the infection within the family, it is only logical to address the mothers of these children. They are best suited to ensure that their children do not get trachoma by introducing better hygienic practices in their households.

The first trial at the end of 1975 failed completely, although Peter Kok and Erika thought they had prepared it well. According to common practice at the time, they first contacted the key people in the community, the chief, the teachers and the clinic nurse – but not the people themselves. Those appointed to do the actual intervention in their community, giving

Erika with the first two Care Group motivators, Selina Maphorogo and social worker Andrew Radebe, 1976

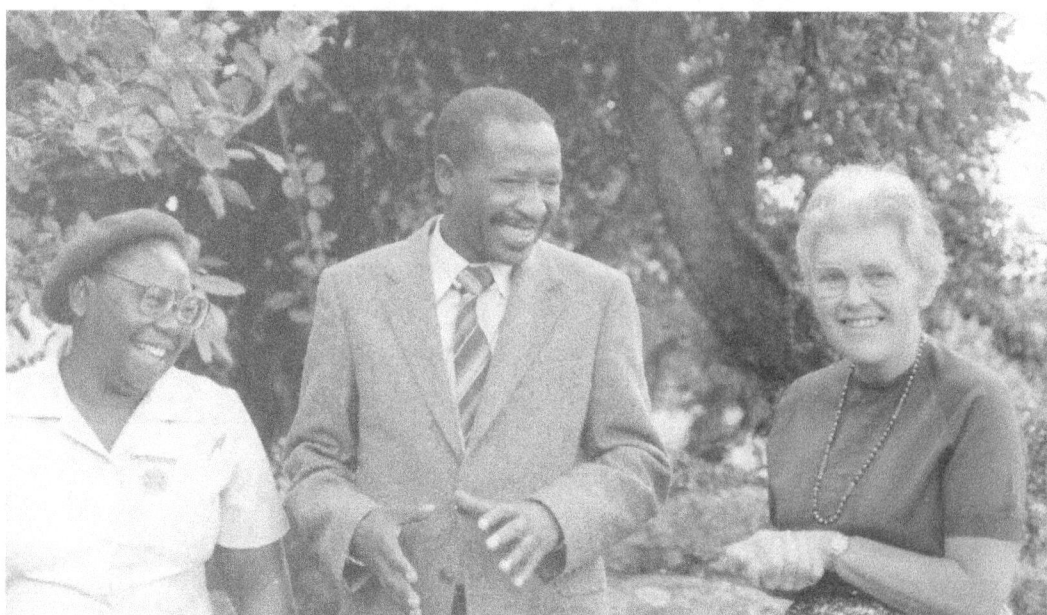

health education and dispensing the eye ointment, were the local women's club. They were snobbish and refused to go to the poorest people who were the most affected by the disease, because they were seen as "dirty people".

A new start was made in three villages, Chavani, Mtsetweni and Nkuzana, this time *with* the people concerned. After long discussions about trachoma, a group of women decided to join the fight against this unnecessary and preventable disease by working as unpaid volunteers. Within weeks, there was a rapid demand for the new project to visit new villages.

This success was largely due to Selina Maphorogo, who became the first Care Group motivator. Erika's Tsonga was not good enough to give health and education lectures to the Care Group women, or lead discussions with them. Selina had already shown remarkable empathy with patients, and Erika therefore chose her as translator. In the beginning there was a social and professional distance between them. Erika was a doctor, and Selina was in the lower ranks of the nursing hierarchy. Over the years of close co-operation, a deep friendship was to grow which lasts until today.

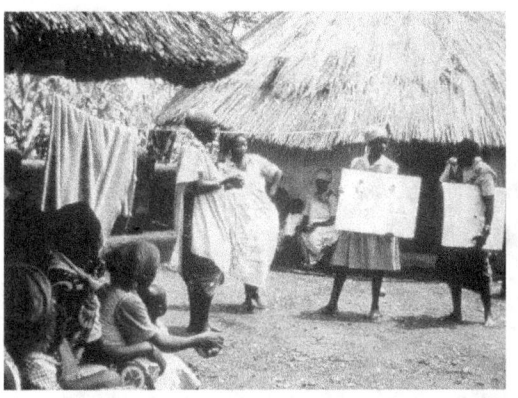
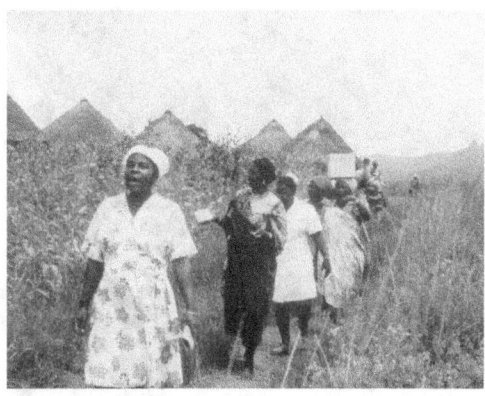

Left:
Care Group members visiting families in their village to advise them about healthy living, 1977

Right:
Care Group members on their way home from a meeting, singing about what they have just learned, 1976

The Care Groups grew fast. Selina said, "We did not do family planning with them! First there were the three groups, then the word spread, and one village after another started. We quickly ran out of eye ointment. Some groups started before the motivators even got to them. We went from three to 27 groups in the first year."

Erika now became responsible for leading and managing a development project that grew into a substantial movement, covering dozens of villages, a responsibility for which she felt she was not fit. And at the same time she felt that she was constantly confronted with higher expectations of her – especially from the motivators – than she felt she could ever fulfil.

The essence of the Care Group Programme at its start was to mobilise local women to form groups and spread their newly acquired knowledge about trachoma within their own area. It was different from other community health projects at the time in that the women worked as groups, and not as individuals. They were regularly visited by their motivator, who was trained by Erika. They would discuss relevant health matters with the motivator who as far as possible let them find their own solution to the problem. The members wore colourful head scarves to distinguish them from other villagers.

Their slogan was, "Cleanliness is the best medicine." This included, among other things, the use of individual face cloths, regular washing of face and hands, building good pit latrines and, where necessary, inserting tetracycline eye ointment. In the past, only trained health personnel had been allowed to insert ointment into eyes. Later, many more health interventions were added, such as child nutrition, vegetable gardening, oral rehydration, and general community development. The work of the Care Groups also came to include informing people about HIV/AIDS, and assisting affected families and orphans.

The great majority of members of the Care Groups are women, but this was not a conscious decision when the project started. Erika says:

> I did not see it from the start as a women's thing. It came later, just automatically, that it was mainly women, and most groups were completely women. There were always some men, and they came especially in connection with the gardening. I was happy when they were involved. Men were never excluded – though in the homelands, there were not many men. Once I was clear, though, about the best way to do something about the spread of trachoma, it was logical to start with the mothers of young children.

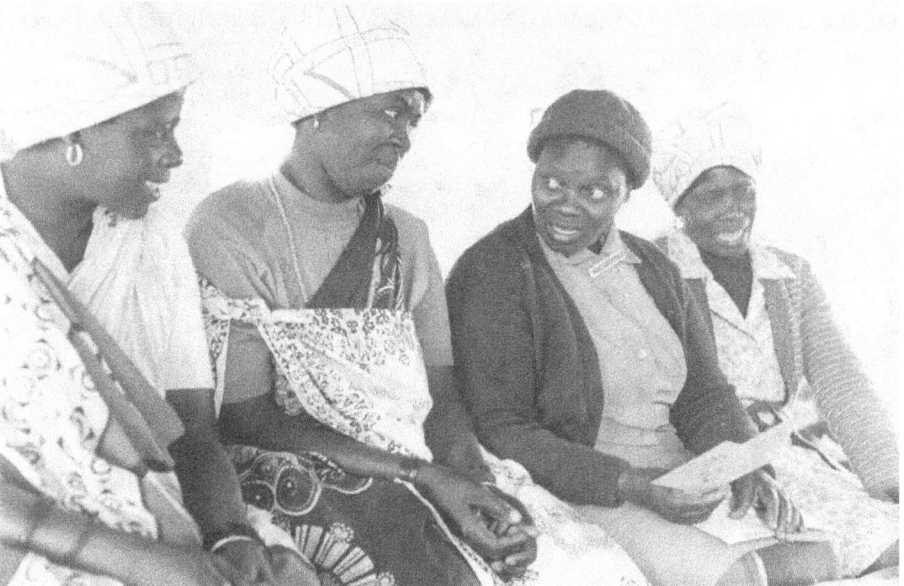

Care Group motivator Florence in a discussion with a group, 1980

When Erika left in 1984, about 10,000 members were organised into some 200 groups in the territories then known as Gazankulu and Venda, which now fall largely under the new provinces of Limpopo and Mpumalanga. This is an unusually large number of people, outside of the church or a political party, to be mobilised in rural areas. This may be due to the forced population removals of the past years which painfully disrupted community life. Erika believes that people were now craving for something where they would get involved in a common aim, as well as having some fun together.

The Care Groups have been written up from the perspective of community-based ophthalmology and community development. *Hanyane: A village struggles for Eye Health* tells the story of a village addressing trachoma and other health issues. The second book, *The Community is my University*, is a collaboration between Erika and Selina Maphorogo, a key actor in the story of the Care Groups, and their senior motivator.

This chapter is about Erika herself, and her role. The core question in it is, how did she manage the work? She says often that she had no choice; that she simply had to get on with it. She points out that she was already quite well known locally, having been at the hospital for 20 years before the Care Groups started. But it was a marginalised and neglected area of South Africa, and she was working with African women who were subjected to and by patriarchal structures, their blackness, and their limited rights. Furthermore, she was in a hospital based mostly on the predominant narrow curative model of health, within a church which overall had a conservative and paternalistic approach to African communities. Any grassroots organising drew the attention of the state security police. This was not the mythical and idyllic "Africa" of some European imaginations: it could be a tough, conflicted and scary place.

So, how did she start the project? How did she develop the leadership role? Where did she learn this different approach to community health care? Where did her support come from? What gave her courage to continue? What were the main barriers to the work? On reflection, what does she think the main achievements have been? And what would she have done differently if she were to start all over again?

Leadership and being a leader

According to Erika:

> Right from my first studies of biology, I have been a good team worker. I am not a good leader. But in Africa, I had to be a leader – in the laboratory, in the hospital as the eye specialist, and in the Care Groups. I was always being challenged to do things for which I was not trained, and which were beyond my capacity, and this was against my character. I realised I was not a leader by nature. I was always happier in a team, not alone guiding people.

Yet it must be said that she created her own role as pioneer-leader for the Care Groups. She thought that it might run according to a perfect plan, but how wrong she was! It was clear early on that the "perfect project" was not going to work, and she had continually to adapt herself, to be flexible, according to the reality of the villagers and Care Group members. And she has come to realise that it was an advantage that she was not trained in community development, and could not have a structured plan. She had to be flexible, adapt herself, go at the pace of the people, allowing the project constantly to change in ways she did not have in mind when the project started. In this, she relied profoundly on the knowledge, insights and skills of Selina Maphorogo.

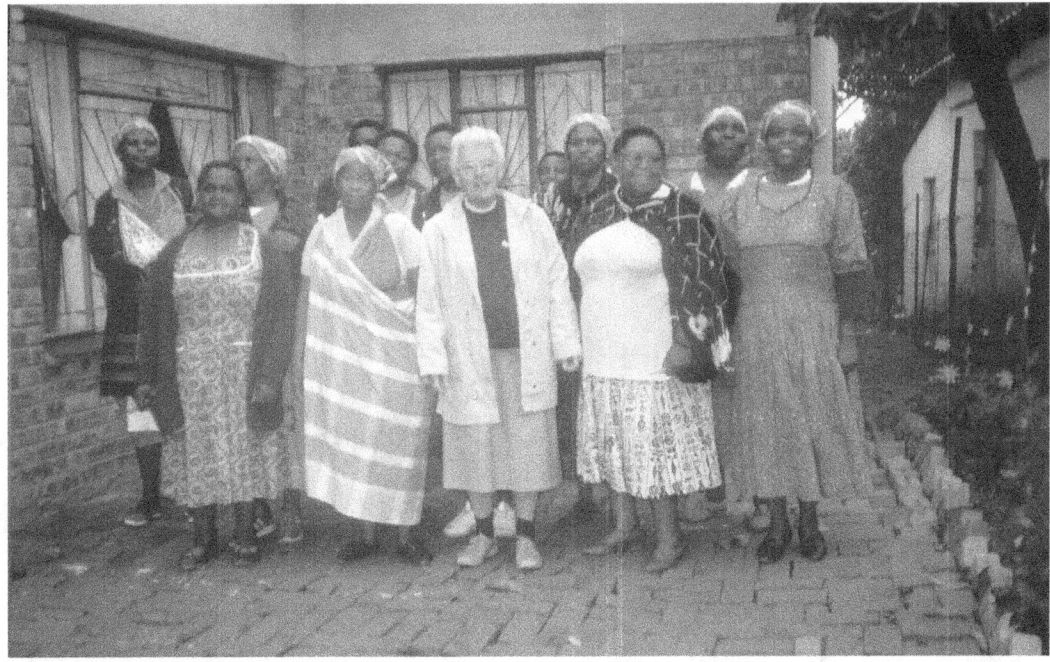

On a visit to Elim in 1996, Erika attended a workshop of the Care Group Top Executive

Health education based on what people know

Both books, *Hanyane* and *The Community is my University* have many examples of how problems in the Care Groups were solved by building on what Care Group members already knew. This differs completely from conventional medical practice that assumes that lay people, in this case villagers, know nothing and that one has to teach them everything. Erika came to be a "true believer" in indigenous knowledge:

> In health education, I had to learn that it did not go the way I thought it would. It is not enough to tell the people. You must go at the pace of the people. They have first to internalise and convince themselves. That's why Selina was so good. In *The Community is my University* Selina relates how she learned to do health education properly, by starting with existing knowledge, and letting people themselves become aware of the problems, and then learning to solve the problems with their own ideas.

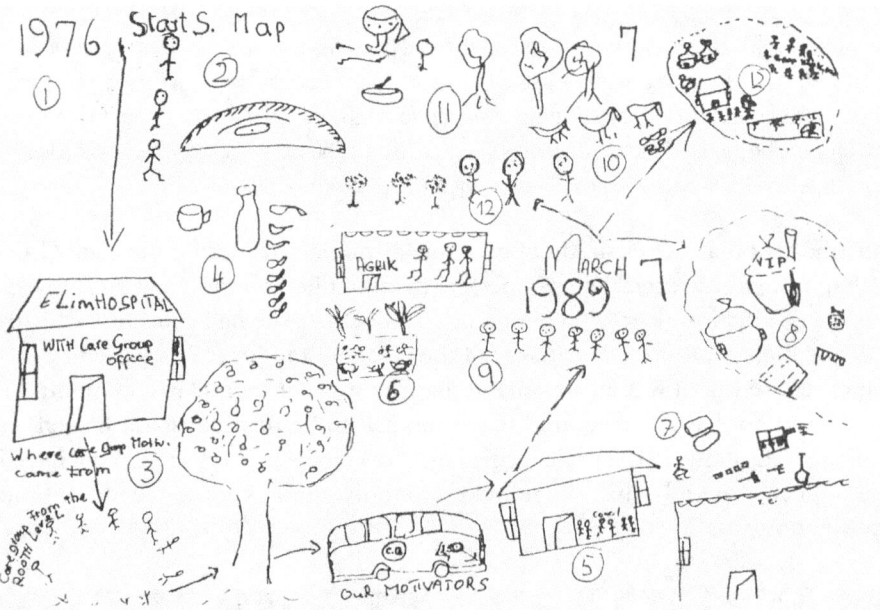

An example of a Care Group's self-evaluation through "social mapping", 1994

> So many things we did turned out to be different from my idea of what should happen, but because they were the members' own ideas, they actually applied them. If I had suggested doing something they would have thought, "This is the doctor's business, it belongs to the hospital, not to us". I would not have been credible because I had running water and electricity in my home. If they wanted to improve their own environment, and solve problems with their own means, they would do it in a way that was practical for them. This is also the reason why I chose nursing assistants rather than fully trained nurses as motivators. The assistants are much closer to the people.

The holistic and practical approach is required if there is to be a lasting impact on health – it requires a change in the professionals, even more than in the people they are serving:

> I always say that an ophthalmologist in a rural area has to know how to build a toilet! You can't just be a single minded ophthalmologist, only doing your medical job, because it is an all-round business. It was very exciting for me to learn methods of community development. I got to learn a lot of things – how to make toilets, and mud stoves, and how to make vegetable driers, instead of having the vegetables drying too slowly and getting rain on them. We also made "fridges",

> with a box with a tray of water on top, and a cloth on both sides. With evaporation this cooled the inside, so that people in the villages, such as diabetics, could keep the insulin cool. These things were very interesting for me.

It is clear that Erika derives a lot of excitement and joy from what was for her a new approach. One senses that perhaps this is where the scientist, the creative artist and the person who loves technology came together in harmony. She also got great enjoyment from the ability of villagers to shape their own environment. In the early 1980s, when Care Groups were learning about building mud stoves, some of them started engraving the drying mud with the name "Ellerine's". This was a large furniture retail store, selling furniture which few local people could afford, and there was a delicious irony in the way the villagers used the store name to take "ownership" of their mud stoves, as if to say, "I can't afford an electric stove, so now you can see this mud stove is my big electric stove!"

Erika recalls:

> There was a good Care Group at Riverplaats. People started with the stoves in the kitchen hut, then made all their furniture. There was a lot of imagination: even a bed made of mud! So this became modern architecture. Then it seems that Ellerine's objected. They told the Care Groups that they were not allowed to continue writing the brand name on the stoves!

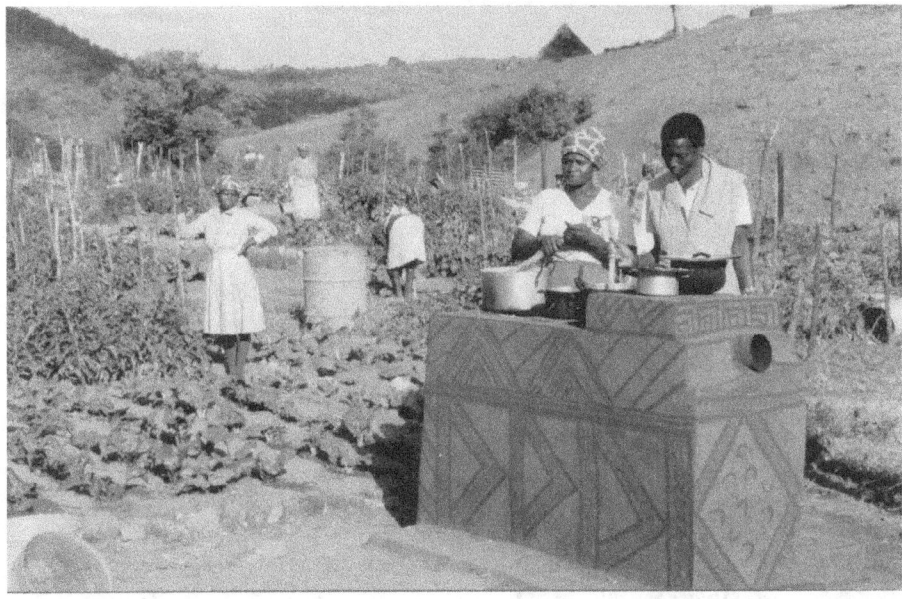

Demonstration mud stove in the communal garden in Riverplaats, ca. 1980

A great endorsement for the Care Group approach to health education came later from her nephew Luke. Erika recalls:

> When we wrote *Hanyane*, I gave it to Luke to read. He is a primary school teacher, and he said that the educational methods in *Hanyane* were better than those we have in the schools in Switzerland!

Managing time and people

Community development is meant to work "at the pace of the community". However, many who have control over the projects work according to a strict time frame, and have to prove to funding bodies that they have achieved "results". The Care Groups started within the hospital, which of course had its own rules and regulations, and the project was partly funded from external sources. Erika, as leader, had to manage and negotiate complex relationships and conflicting expectations, inside and outside the project.

As recorded in *The Community is my University*, Selina felt she was thrown in at the deep end, and she did not realise at first that Erika was right there in the deep end with her! Erika struggled to find her own place with the motivators. She appointed some people, towards the beginning, who were not suitable. Selina stood out as one who would worry about the project after hours, trying to use her own initiative to solve problems. Even she, however, became demoralised at times to see that the matrons and her fellow nursing assistants did not regard what she was doing as real work. Erika feared Selina might leave the project:

> I was scared that one day she would say, "No, that's enough! I want to go back to the ward!" I told her that it was not an easy situation for me either. But the great difference between me and her was that I was doing it because I wanted to do it, whereas she did it because I told her to do it. It was not of her own free will.

Like Selina, some other motivators also felt they were not understood or accepted by their peers. "What a strange thing this is that you are doing, talking to people in the community", hospital nursing assistants would say to them. At the same time, many worked so passively and so slowly, that it sometimes frustrated Erika:

> I wanted them to use their own initiative in finding out about technologies, and ways of adult education. I had to learn that many came from very remote rural areas, where they did not have the inputs that the people in town have. For them, the world they were used to had always been like that, and most of them did not think of ways of doing otherwise. I was disappointed in the motivators. I expected them to be as enthusiastic as I was, and not to watch the clock, but to put their whole person into the work. But for them – apart from Selina – it was just a job. This was understandable, because they needed a job.

> The motivators started to complain about their long working hours, and their poor salaries. I tried to persuade Pierre Jaques about the need for higher salaries, but the health department was bound to grade nursing assistants according to set pay scales, and they could not change that. It was a continual fight for me to convince hospital management that motivators are more

Overhead projector transparencies, used by Erika in teaching in the STI

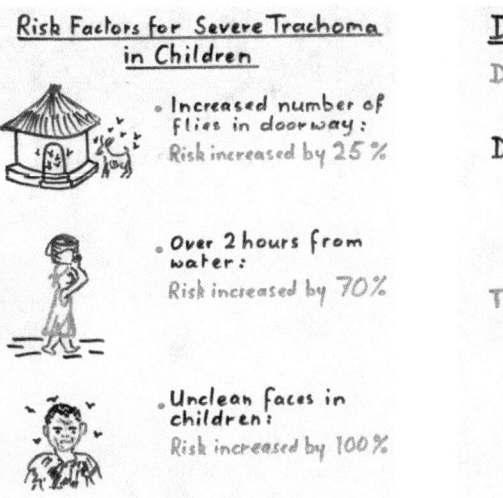
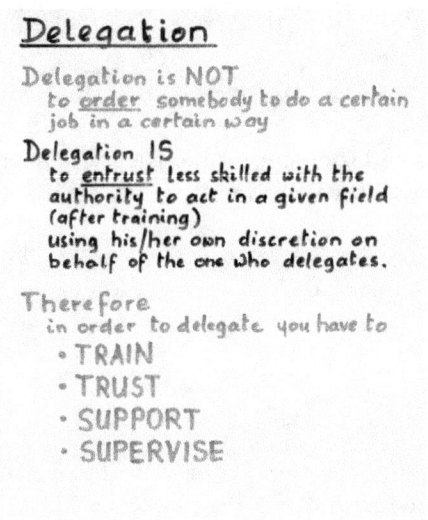

than hospital assistant nurses, and that they are able to think independently, are not ignorant, and do not need step-by-step instructions.

Erika wonders whether her medical training may have limited the potential of the motivators to grow:

> As far as my work was concerned, I did give the motivators too little responsibility – for example in the project's financial matters, which I kept under my own control. We had very limited finance during the first years. It was enough to cover the note pads and pencils for the women in the groups, and a little to cover the eye ointment. I also never spoke to the motivators about project finance. This would, however, have been a good idea – to show them what such a project costs.
>
> Carel IJsselmuiden, my successor, was of the opinion that I used to visit the groups too often. I do not agree, however. I did go to the groups often in the beginning, until Selina took them over herself. I sometimes went to observe the motivators, as they were trained to work in hospitals, not for their work in villages. I went to observe and to give some elementary tips – for example, not to turn one's back to the women while demonstrating something but to make sure that all could see what was being demonstrated.
>
> What Carel did much better than me was to work intensively with the motivators to enable them to stand their ground with their superiors regarding their opinions as to what was important, and when necessary to disagree with them. This naturally angered the matrons, who claimed it was "cheeky behaviour".

Finding support

As the project continued, Erika had to spend a lot of time and energy in the hospital explaining what the point of the Care Groups was, and how the motivators would need support in their work – and especially that the motivators' times of work needed to be dictated by the everyday rhythm and needs of village life, and not by those of the hospital itself. She did not get much support in this from the matrons or the hospital staff in general, apart from superintendent Pierre Jaques, and from Peter Kok while he was in Elim, and some of the Dutch colleagues.

Erika said:

> Other doctors did not as a rule understand what we were doing. They complained that we were gallivanting around while they were doing the real work in the hospital. They were only interested in the Care Groups when they wanted to make demands of them, when they needed help with their research.

However, there were people who encouraged her work:

> Tiakeni was a remarkable craft development project nearby, with a clear radical political position, and its director Rob Collins was very supportive.
>
> There was a time, in about 1981 and 1982, when everyone seemed to have lost their enthusiasm. Care Groups members stopped coming; the motivators brought nothing new. I thought I was doing it all wrong. Pam Spencer, a physiotherapist working in Elim, supported me a lot at that time.

There was seldom outright hostility, from either the hospital or from the Department of Health. Erika experienced a reaction that was perhaps worse than outright hostility:

> I was not opposed by them, but I got no support from them. This was like coming up against a wall – a wall not made of bricks, but of cotton wool.

Voluntary work

"Community involvement", on a voluntary basis, is of enormous value in community development. From the onset the Care Group project was conceived as voluntary work done by its members. The motivators were paid to do their work, but the group members themselves were unpaid. Is this a reasonable expectation of poor women who needed some source of income, in an area with very few paid employment opportunities for women? On a few occasions, Selina had to respond to requests for payment from members. Erika remembers:

> At the beginning, a few groups demanded to be paid. Selina explained to the women that their own families would profit from the voluntary work. Later on some members realised that they saved a lot of money as they did not need to take the children to the clinic, which cost money every time. They saved through harvesting their own vegetables from their gardens; they could produce their own soap, and so on.

Erika feels that one has to be aware of the different social contexts of Europe and rural South Africa. In Europe, people may be able to do voluntary work at times of their lives when they do not need to earn full-time. In a poor society, she pointed out, time is money and people need to do something productive, either growing things or earning money.

She said:

> I deeply admire the way that all the groups, in such a large area, continue to work without payment. Although the Care Groups only work as a group when they have time, they could choose to use this time for themselves by working in a paid job, if one were available – though there are very few paid employment opportunities for women in the area served by the Care Groups. A further drain on the women's time is the HIV/AIDS pandemic, which is placing a heavy burden of responsibility on them for caring for sick household members.

The Care Groups and the church

Erika's main working area was Gazankulu, where most churches had been established in the past by Swiss missionaries. However, as far as support for community action from the church was concerned, Erika was greatly disappointed:

> When I started the Care Groups, the *Département Missionaire (DM)* in Lausanne was not interested. They did not support us financially. It was not a church programme, as I wanted to be completely neutral. It was only later, when I was already retired, that the Care Groups came to be seen as a positive project of the church. This was to the advantage of the Care Groups. Since then it has been a project of the *DM*, and they support the Care Groups together on a franc for franc basis with the Swiss Government Development Fund paying half, and the mission half. But when I was there, there was little interest from the church.

A principle of the Care Groups, and supposedly in all community development, is that the will of local people is paramount, and their own reality and traditions must be respected. But why then was it that especially in the villages in which the church had been most actively involved, people were reluctant to start their own Care Groups? Erika's opinion was that:

> In the beginning, the mission certainly "mothered" the "poor black people", and the older missionaries in my time still continued in this vein. This image tends to remain in the minds of outsiders, although this is no longer the case. One now works with the people and not for them.

Both Erika and her successor Carel IJsselmuiden feel that some of the church's approach and activities lead to the creation of dependence, to a passive attitude in the villages that the church will sort out their problems, and that they do not need to take action themselves. Erika and Selina have both observed that even within their own church, there are barriers to helping those outside the church:

> We had difficulties with church members in the beginning. Before I started the Care Groups, some of our women's church groups, the *Vamanana*, asked me to give them talks about high blood pressure and eye health. I realised later that they did not spread their knowledge to others. They kept it to themselves. And one of the last communities to join the Care Groups was Elim. Around Elim there are many educated people, who feel that they know everything. This was also the case elsewhere where churches had been active for a long time.

How did Erika get away from paternalism, which often also coincides with a form of racism? And what if the paternalism of the church coincides with the hierarchical power system of the medical profession? Erika thinks that at the beginning, she was not less racist and paternalistic than others in her missionary community:

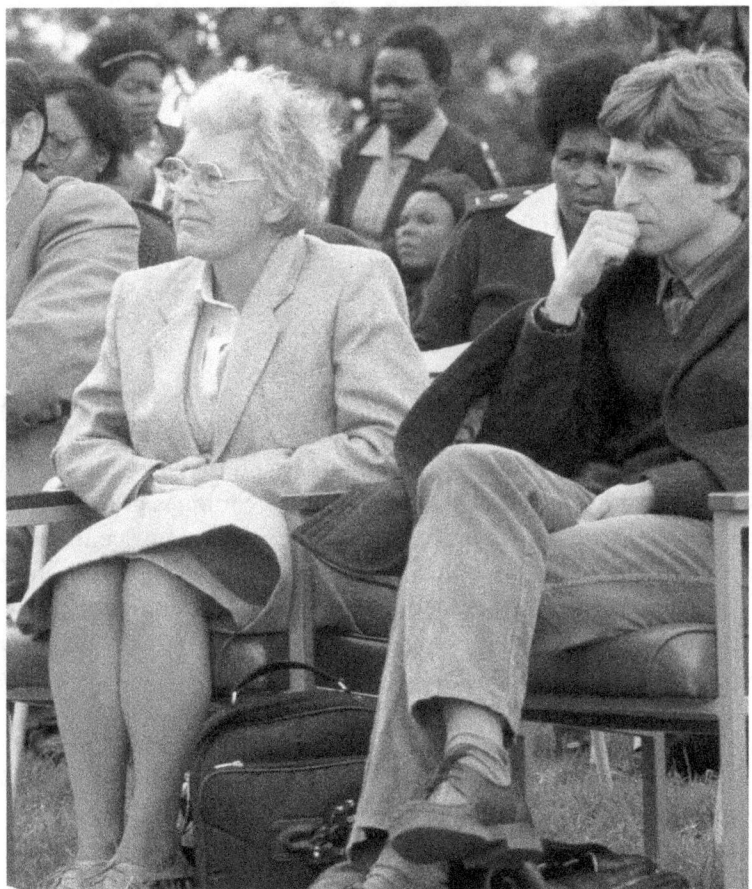

Erika with her successor Carel IJsselmuiden at a farewell event organised by the Venda Care groups, 1984

As a doctor, you were trained to think and behave "top down". It was your job to prevent and to cure. However, as a Christian, I do not think I was a fanatic. And as a middle class person, I was not a snob. But still, I have asked myself whether I should have been so completely neutral, or should I have had more political involvement? Or been more religious, and developed the movement as a specifically Christian group? But neither political involvement nor a religious basis would have been appropriate for the Care Groups. For me, even if I had based the work on Christian grounds I would not have said the Care Groups were only for Christians. As a Christian, it was clear to me that they should be open for everybody.

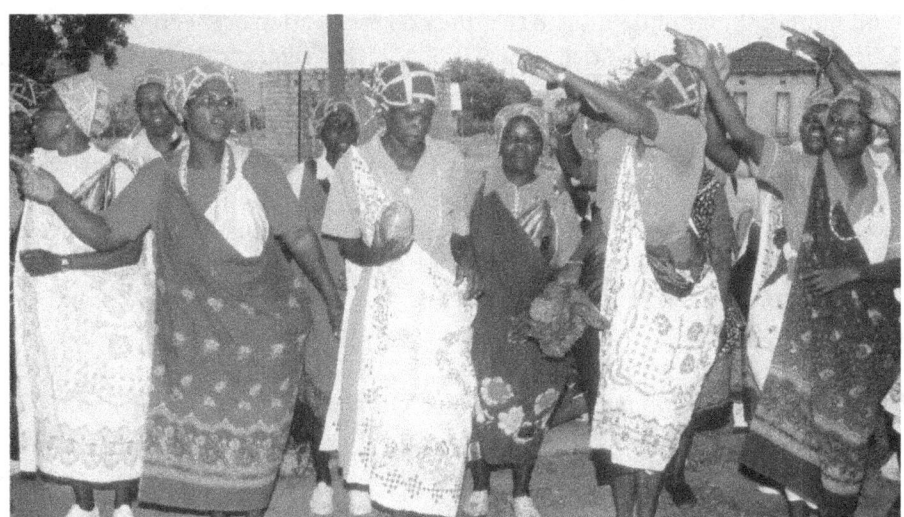

A Care Group demonstrating what is needed for good nutrition by singing and dancing (photo by M.-A. Gneist, ca. 2000)

This open and inclusive approach of Erika's was at odds with the approach of an American evangelical doctor at nearby Acornhoek, who visited Elim after the Care Groups had been going for two or three years. He had started women's groups, doing toilet building, and he was doing this only for Christians, and only those who were members of his church. He visited the Care Groups, who always welcomed a visitor by dancing and beating their drums. This doctor was shocked, called the Care Groups "heathen dancers", and left. This was given by Erika as a bad example of an exclusive church-based approach that sets itself up as a model for what is good, while disrespecting local culture and hospitality.

The repressive political environment

The year that the Care Groups started, 1976, was the year that marked the beginning of the end of apartheid South Africa. School uprisings saw the youth take on the might of the state, and the police brutality was visible through the international media. The apartheid government and its security apparatus developed new techniques of repression, reaching deep into rural areas. In rural development projects, there was little place to hide. As the situation got more serious, observation posts were set up in rural areas and townships to catch anti-apartheid activists. They created great uncertainty: no-one knew if they were being watched, and no-one knew if they were in or out of danger. It was worst in rural areas, where everybody knows everyone else, at least by name and location. It was not possible to be anonymous.

Community development leaders such as Erika are always faced with the question of how to engage with politics. Some see community development as a vehicle for political struggle; others refuse to engage politically at all. The position of leaders has implications for others – in this case, for the literally thousands of Care Group members who had mobilised around eye care.

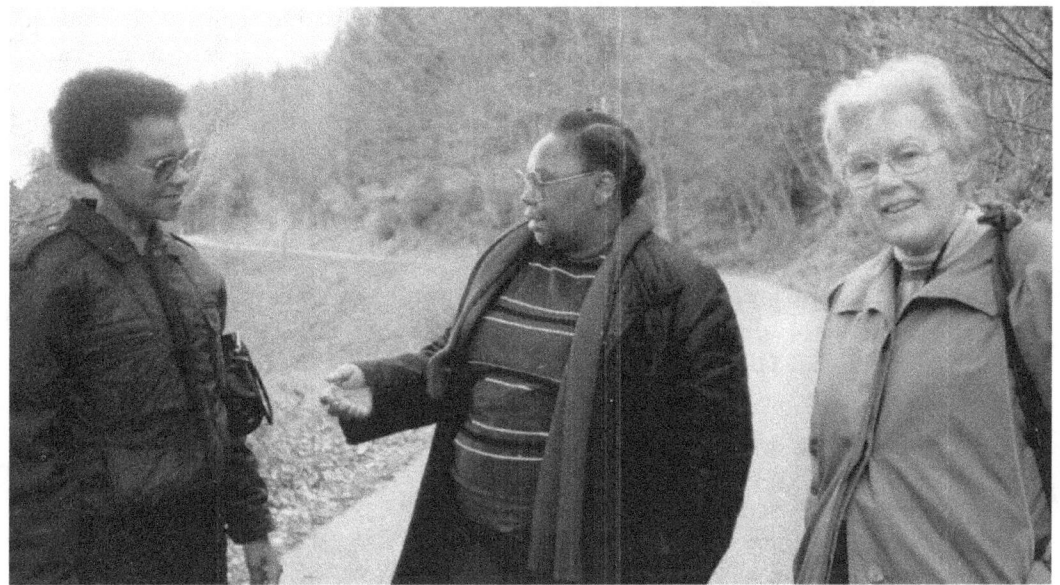

Mamphela Ramphele, Selina and Erika in the Black Forest (Germany), just over the border from Basel, 1989

One day in 1983 Erika got a surprise visit from a man who pretended he was a social worker who wanted to return to Gazankulu to work. This was directly after Erika had seen anti-apartheid visitors from the USA. Their itinerary had included visiting Dr Mamphela Ramphele, the well-known anti-apartheid activist who was forced through political legislation to reside in the local area – she was a "banned" person. The man wanted a list of Care Group members, saying it was in connection with his work with the Gazankulu health department. During the conversation Erika came to realise that he was from the security police. Erika gave him a minimum of information, and not the list of members, and superintendent Pierre Jaques told him to go away. Erika then realised how, "Development is itself suspicious. People are not meant to think and act independently".

Later on, Erika discussed the issue of political engagement with Dr Ramphele

> I asked Mamphela whether I should have been more political with the Care Groups. She felt that, in a case like this where the women have come together not as an anti-apartheid movement, but to learn something about health, you could not get them involved in an anti-apartheid movement, unless they chose to do this themselves. If anyone had been caught, without knowing why, and had been tortured...! This you couldn't do.

On looking back, Erika feels she was right. She also frankly admits she would not have had the courage to resist more openly. And she was confident that political consciousness would grow automatically through their health work, which included training in awareness and problem-solving. About six months after the ANC came to power in 1994, Selina phoned Erika:

> With her tongue in her cheek – I could see this on the phone! – Selina said, "It is much more difficult now working with women. They want to know everything about why we do what we do! They do not say 'yes' so easily any more!"

Ubuntu: People are a gold mine

The Care Groups were one of a number of community health projects that emerged during the late 1970s. Some were influenced by the spreading information about primary health care and the Alma Ata Conference; others had a more explicitly anti-apartheid framework which included using primary health care as a basis for political mobilisation. I think that a number of things made this particular project unique. There was organisation of grassroots rural women in groups on a fairly large scale, rather than health workers visiting only on a household basis. The project was based in a hospital, which gave it some protection and institutional stability, but Erika actually managed to negotiate a fair amount of flexibility in how it operated. This flexibility was then dedicated to trying to develop basic values of community development, such as listening carefully and building direction slowly.

Remarkably, the Care Groups have now been operating for over 30 years, surviving the political transition, and have adjusted their work to include dealing with HIV and AIDS. For this final section on the Care Groups, Erika was asked to look back, with the wisdom of hindsight, and give us her current perspectives on the project and her views about what might happen in the future:

> Like other issues of my 32 years in South Africa, I understood much of it better when looking at it from the outside. I would act differently if I had a chance to start all over again. One question I would approach differently would be how to start such a new venture. As I mentioned earlier on, the Care Group motivators had a tough time when dealing with the matrons or their peers in the hospital. Now, very late, I realise that without being aware of it, I asked too much of them at several levels. Firstly, my concept of community involvement was unknown in the community health teaching of the time. Secondly, community health was regarded as communist in South Africa. Thirdly, the motivators were pushed completely untrained into the difficult task of transforming my goals and health messages into a community process. No wonder the matrons who were responsible for the work done by nursing assistants did not understand what was going on. Possibly it would have helped if I had included all the key people in the hospital when planning the project.

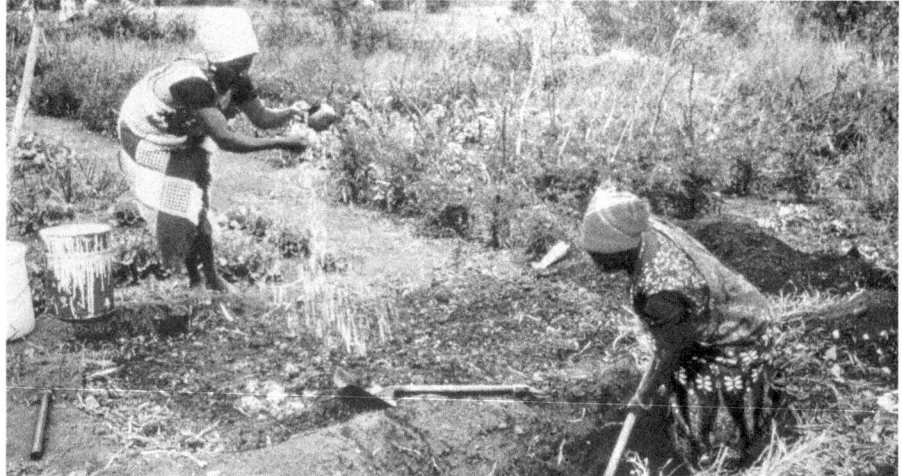

Care Group members in Riverplaats prepare beds for "Deep Trench" vegetable gardening, 1976

> Although the motivators did not tell me, I think they were often unhappy with my attempted leadership. My problem was that I knew exactly, in theory, what I should do, but I was not able to act accordingly and in a positive way. But I know too that as a whole I did not fare too badly. Selina told me often that in contrast to other doctors I always shared my knowledge with the motivators. At the time of the farewell celebrations in 1984, my sister-in-law asked Selina what the Care Groups were saying about my leaving, and she replied, "When they are worried about their future without Dr Sutter, I tell them that we motivators have picked everything out of her brain and put it in our brains, so much that when she flies back to Switzerland, she will be quite light."

> At the time of my retirement people often expressed their doubts about the future of the project, given that I was leaving it to the local black people. This was a typical reaction of Europeans with their superiority complex. My experience was different. While most motivators were also worried about my leaving, Selina said, "This is a challenge for us. We shall show you that we can do it." With this statement in my heart, I could return home with confidence. In my view my greatest achievement was that I became superfluous to the project.

Erika asked me for my own view of her contribution to the project. She has already reflected openly on her own strengths and weaknesses, and I agree with most of her views. I have a few things to add that come from my friendship with her and from my contact with the project over the years. Erika has a deep belief in the African idea of *ubuntu* which means "people are only people through or with other people". She states many a time in this book that she only achieved what she did through being with other people. It is also the case, though, that she often took risks, making herself unpopular, fighting for principles about how the project should operate, in a way that could potentially have alienated her in the remote community in which she lived and worked. She was single-minded and enduring, and in my view sometimes borderline subversive in this, in the best interests of the people in the projects.

Another way in which the project was different from others was in the survey at the start of the project. This demonstrated that the current practice of reaching out to school children was wrong, and that her intervention had to be with young mothers in households, and this scientific foundation was a good weapon in her battle against the approach of the Council for the Blind. She knew from the survey how to start, and she followed this up with a degree of attention to monitoring and evaluation that made the project quite unique at the time.

I think that her belief in *ubuntu* is and was supplemented by other remarkable qualities which were essential to the development of the project. Erika has a fundamental curiosity about the world: about how the laws of nature work, and about how these are understood differently by people from different cultures. Without this, and if she were a more typical or ordinary medical doctor, she might not have given Selina so much time and space to work with the motivators and the members of the Care Groups in trying to develop an authentic local practice of community development.

Many projects fail when leaders move on too early, perhaps because funding runs out, or the younger leader wants to move on to the next rung in a career ladder. Erika, by contrast, started the Care Groups at a mature age, when she was known in the community, and intending to stay to retirement age, which gave her eight years in the Care Groups.

What, then, about Erika's views on the future of the Care Groups?

> People ask me whether the Care Groups will continue with changing times. I think something will continue in some way or other, at least as long as the present members are still here. These women are strong and have withstood many difficult times where they have been left in the lurch. They have internalised the issues of health and village development and over the more than thirty years of the project's existence they have taken ownership of it. They know now where to go when they need more information, and their communities trust them now and come to them when they need advice. They have developed a lasting health awareness, and better hygiene has become the norm.
>
> Some factors might get in the way of their continuing. The Groups may decide that they have already achieved all that they set out to do. It could also be that, with the generation change,

the young women will decide that they want to be paid as Care Group members. Also, much will depend on what the national and the provincial services decide about the place of and support for such community-based health initiatives. I am also aware that the new global developments may change a society, even this remote rural one, quite radically.

However, even if the groups stop functioning, it was worthwhile, and it is an achievement in itself that they lasted so long. Their imprint is still there. And they have become a fixed feature of village life. I have seen a change in the attitudes of these rural women beyond my expectations. They have found their self-confidence and dignity as women. This is real empowerment, and this is more important than better health. And it is not only the women who have changed, but their whole community. Health awareness is now the norm, and this is even recognised by the authorities, who told me that in places where Care Groups are active, new interventions can easily be introduced.

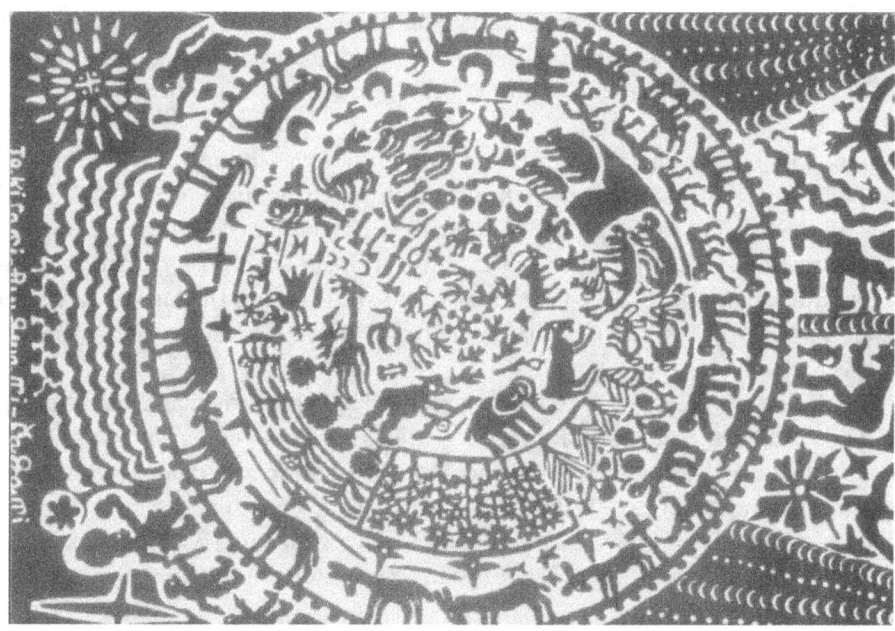

"Wisdom circle" or circle of life (an expression of ubuntu). Woodcut by the artist and "prophet" Jackson Hlungwane in Mbokota.

It was a great enrichment for me that, through the mediation of Selina, I started to understand the rural people better. I felt their great warmth, their inner strength which enabled them to maintain their happy mood, laughter and music in the midst of grinding poverty. I enjoyed their generous hospitality and felt accepted by them and belonged to them. This was confirmed on one of my visits to South Africa from Switzerland. One of the Care Group members presented me with a wonderful praise poem, something they usually only offer to important people of their community, such as village chiefs.

A PRAISE POEM FOR DR SUTTER
By K.M. Hlongwane, Malamulele[1]

Hoyo, Hoyooo
Welcome among us all, our dear eye-doctor,
You who taught us the rules of true and careful growth,
Through sincere devotion to all our people,
You invented for us all kinds of new foodstuffs.
We saw that you differed from "get-rich" other whites.

You hailed from Switzerland, a Gospel-source for us.
When your thoughts visit us, they give you itchy feet.
You made us rub the dirt from our sleepy eyes;
If only we could find other doctors like you.

Go well, dear Erika, Grandma to our teams,
We shall remember you, we your true grandchildren.
Every time they ponder your labours in their midst,
All mothers and fathers try to emulate you,
And make your great talent bear fruit for them also.
Your work stands before them like a shining mirror.

We call you "Topisa", the one who stops the diseases;
We are the grateful heirs of the famous Care Groups,
Unknown in other lands.
People flock to see them with wonder and envy.
The whole country will soon come here to learn and grow.
May the good Lord grant you many more days on earth.

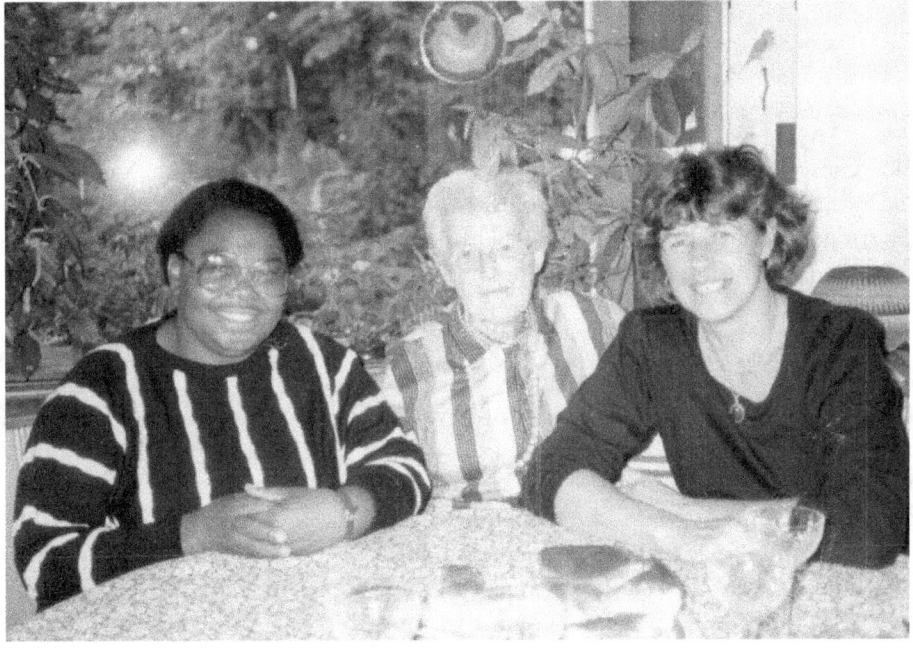

Selina, Erika und Frances Lund in Basel, 1989

Endnote

1   Translated from the original Tsonga by Theo Schneider, 26.02.96.

VIII Retirement and the return to Basel

Preparations for retirement

In 1984, Erika decided to retire at the age of 67. Thoughts about where to spend the final phase of her life had occupied her mind for at least three years, and it was now clear to her that returning to Basel would be best, rather than remaining in South Africa. In 1981 she had been in Basel, undergoing surgery for glaucoma for the first time, in the Basel Eye Hospital. Lying in the hospital bed she let herself be taken care of, and experienced just how precious the visits of her family were. Even though she had many dear friends in South Africa, wouldn't she miss this closeness with her family as she got old? In Basel, she felt as though she belonged. But how would she feel as an unmarried missionary woman remaining in Elim? Erika reflected on one such *"demoiselle missionnaire"*:

> She stayed there for a long time and became a real burden for us, in particular for her best friend, Gabrielle Guy, who had to go to her every weekend and was very tied down as a result. Many retired missionaries did stay in the country in which they had served, but they had children close by who had also settled there. In earlier times, a single person would have been adopted into the "missionary family". But the "missionary family" had shrunk significantly. I was virtually the last one who had chosen to serve until I was old enough to retire.

So Erika realised that there would be no one in Elim to care for her as she grew old. She was also not interested in living in white South Africa, and it was doubtful that the government would permit her to live in a "homeland" without working there. After considering all of this, Erika resolved to return to Switzerland.

Who would be Erika's successor?

The search for a successor in Elim was now a priority. A good solution for the management of the Eye Hospital was no problem; Dr Pius Bucher, a colleague of Erika's for the last six months, was prepared to assume the responsibility. However, finding the right person to take over the Care Groups proved to be difficult. In order to aid the search, in 1983 a weekend workshop on community health care was organised, to which selected individuals from all over South Africa were invited. It took place in the Ben Lavin Game Reserve, a small game park just 15 kilometres from Elim, where it was possible to arrange shared accommodation for mixed-race groups. The event resulted in three fascinating days, positive feedback, and many new contacts and connections – in particular with Frances Lund from Durban, whose friendship has continued to this day, including involvement with the present book. Unfortunately, no one volunteered to take over the Care Groups. But finally a Dutch doctor, Carel IJsselmuiden, expressed interest and agreed to succeed Erika in this capacity.

Initial preparations for retirement

"The first couple of years back home will be really tough!" Erika was told by someone reflecting on their own experience. She hoped to counteract this, so she put out her feelers in advance of her return home, looking to find something meaningful to do after retirement that would draw on her experience and knowledge:

Already during my vacation in 1981, I got in touch with the Swiss Tropical Institute in Basel (now the Swiss Tropical and Public Health Institute), to ask whether they could use me in the courses they had for medical personnel going to the tropics. At the time, Professor Thierry Freyvogel was Director. Towards the end of my work in Elim, I received a letter from Professor Barry Jones in England. He had just founded the International Centre for Eye Health (ICEH) in London, and wrote to me about some papers I'd written together with Ron Ballard. He suggested that only "angels" could bring a popular movement like the Care Groups to life. I wrote back that there were no angels working here in Elim, just good people like my closest collaborator, Selina Maphorogo, and that I'd be very interested to work at his institute in some small capacity following retirement. It was only later that he remembered that I'd attended his lectures a long time ago when I was working for my Diploma in Ophthalmology in London. The result was that I became a lecturer in these London courses myself.

At very short notice, in the midst of her final weeks in Elim, Erika received a request to give two presentations at a symposium in London, jointly organised by the WHO and the ICEH. While she was visiting Europe, Erika had the chance to spend a week in Basel and look for a flat.

The grand departure from Elim

In February 1984, Erika's brother Ernst and his wife Gaby came to visit Elim once more. They wanted to share more of Erika's life in Elim, in order to understand her experience in South Africa better, as they would be together a lot in the future. They were joined by friends, another married couple, so it was as a group of five that they travelled around. Erika left the driving to her visitors, as she could no longer drive long distances on account of her poor eyesight. Everyone in Elim had been waiting for Erika's family to arrive before beginning with the farewell festivities. But now the fun could begin:

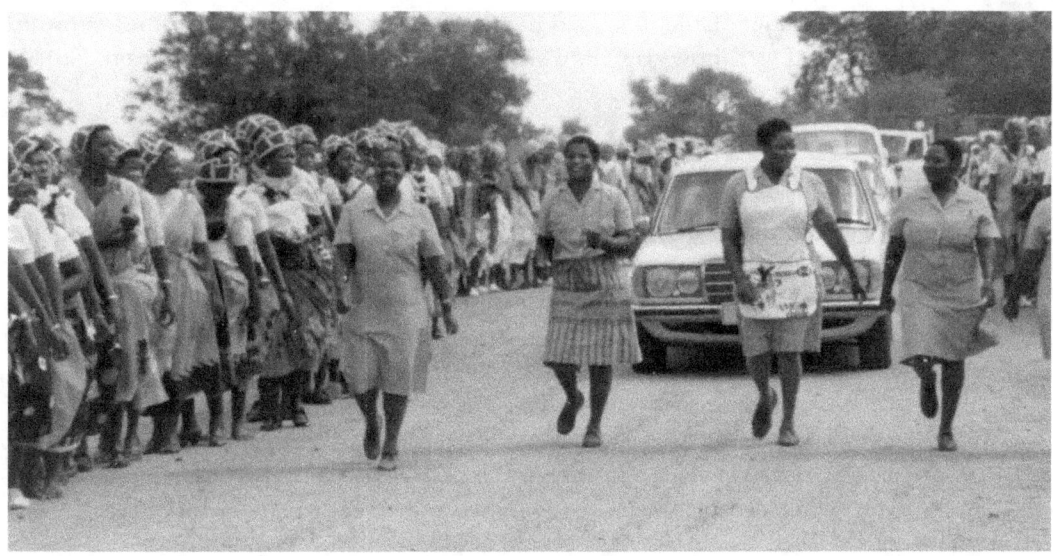

Farewell from the Care Groups at Giyani Show Ground, 1984

The first to fête me were the Care Groups. The celebration took place in Giyani, in the large Agricultural Show Ground. Out of six thousand members, about three thousand women showed up. We travelled there in a hospital station wagon, driven by one of the doctors. When we arrived, we had to wait on the main street and then, together with a delegation from the Gazankulu government, we passed through a long guard of honour formed by the Care Groups until we got to the show ground. I felt like the Queen of England! Everything was fantastically well organised, especially by Selina, who made sure that the groups' presentations didn't go on forever and that there was space here and there for a song or a demonstration. The President of the Elim Care Group, who had previously been a patient of mine, took the occasion to relate the story of a fellow patient on whom I'd performed cataract surgery. After the operation, the patient had absolutely refused to sleep in a bed. She said she couldn't, that her "tribal doctor" had forbidden her to do it. So I had told the nurses to let the patient sleep on a mattress on the floor, which completely calmed her down. That impressed people.

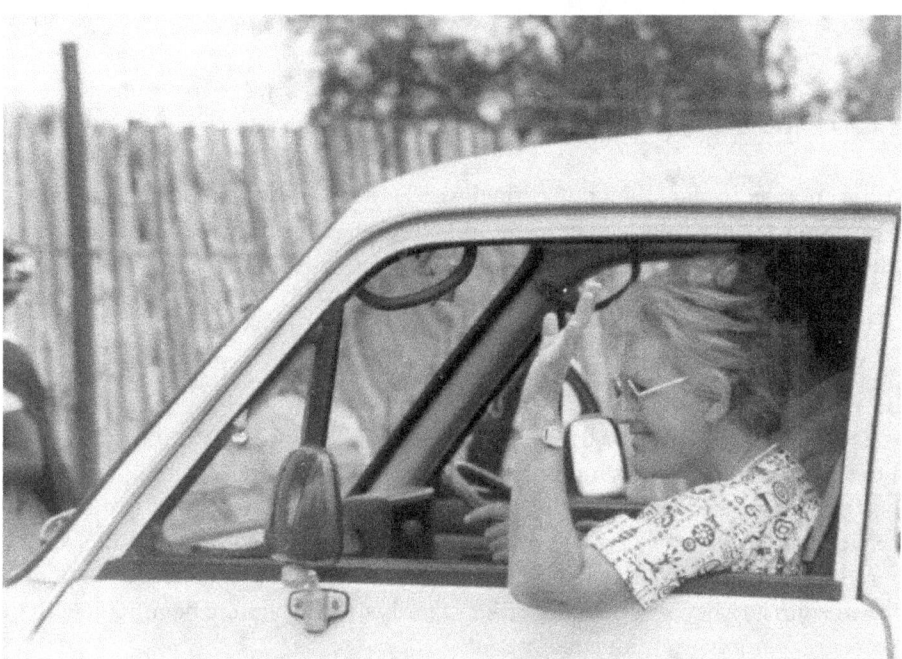

Erika waves "Goodbye" to the Care Groups (feeling like the Queen of England), 1984

At the end of the ceremony, Erika received many gifts. It was her most beautiful farewell. Next came the send-off at Elim Hospital, which was well organised by the Matron. Erika's memories bubbled over:

To start with, the domestic staff sang a song. They were followed by the Care Group motivators. Next, students from the School for Ophthalmic Nursing put on a play about a day in my life. The Sister Tutor played me. She portrayed me greeting the students for the first lesson in the morning, saying to one after another: "You are ...? You are ...? I am sorry, I don't remember your name." Then came a scene where I was shown taking photographs of the Care Groups. I could really see myself in their interpretation. They are keen observers and wonderful actors – it was really delightful. At the end, the medical superintendent, Pierre Jaques, announced a special surprise for me. All of my former students who could make it were there! They appeared in civilian clothes, and I had to greet them. A uniform would have given me some clue as to what hospital they were from, but dressed as they were I couldn't recall their names and was forced to play myself, in a manner of speaking, and ask them each who they were. The audience roared with laughter.

When it was finally time to leave, Erika was picked up from her little home by the Rivoni manager's wife, driving a *camionette* (pickup truck), and taken to Johannesburg. Their path took them past the hospital, where the staff members lined the road from the top down to the Chapel to bid her "Good-bye". The majorette group of the nursing students marched in front of her car to the beat of their drums. Erika, close to tears, could hardly bear it, and before they reached the end of the hospital grounds, she whispered to her driver, "Come on, step on it!"

The return to Basel, and new contacts

With the understanding help of her family, Erika was able to manage her return home to Basel very well. Her new flat in the Neubad area was wonderfully sunny and bright, with plenty of room for treasures brought back from Africa and furniture inherited from her family. It was on the second floor, without a lift, but sprightly Erika was able to cope with the stairs for fourteen more years. In 1988, at the age of eighty-one, she used her remaining strength to move into her present lovely home, with a lift, in the Bachletten district. "I won't be leaving this flat of my own free will," she says with determination.

In the initial period after her return, Erika found herself feeling "pretty uneasy". She suddenly had lots of time to herself, which had never been the case before! Those pesky first two years that she'd heard about were now upon her. One simply had to get used to it inwardly. But Erika wouldn't have been herself if she hadn't take matters into her own hands. She began to look around to see who among her old friends was still about. She only found a handful of friends from her youth, but even after more than thirty years away she was able to reconnect with them almost without missing a beat. "It was as if I'd never left." Among those she rediscovered was Lilly Stählin, a former schoolmate, who lived on the same street and took her to the monthly get-togethers of her old classmates. But in general, Erika found that – unlike in Africa – elderly people here have a tendency to remain within their own established groups, lacking curiosity about new encounters. So it was up to her to approach people herself, and take the first step. It is impressive to learn how Erika built up a new network of contacts:

> There is a women's group belonging to my local church, St. Stephen's, in which I still participate actively. In this group I established long-lasting friendships with Marie-Claire Barth and Margrith Amstutz. Our joint missionary background, in particular, connects Marie-Claire and myself; with Margrith it's our shared botanical interests and many years of long walks together in Splügen. From 1993 to 1999, I took part regularly in courses in "breathing gymnastics" held at an altitude of two thousand metres on Alp Flix in Graubünden. They were organised by Ursula Scherrer, who also became a friend of mine. There was always ample time for hiking during the course; at first, my body struggled with the huge difference in altitude between Basel and Alp Flix, but I learned to bridge the difference by staying for a time in Splügen, at fifteen hundred metres, before proceeding to Alp Flix.
>
> Not long after I got back to Basel, Vreni Schneider, secretary of the Swiss Mission in South Africa within the umbrella organisation Kooperation Evanglische Kirchen und Missionen (KEM), invited me for a discussion in the headquarters of the Basel Mission. From then on, I was frequently in and out of the Mission House. One day, I met Waltraud Haas there, and she told me about the South Africa group of the Women's Association of the Swiss Evangelical Churches. The group published worksheets based on personal accounts from people and groups in South Africa who had suffered because of their resistance to apartheid. Waltraud asked for my help with the number that was just coming out, which was on child labour. Afterwards, I went on working with the group, until 1994. In this group, I got to know Dorothea Rüsch, and through her, I also got to know about movements concerned with the environment and with fair trade. In those days, people chuckled dismissively about such groups. Dorothy's dedication in sticking to her principles was and is an example to me to this day, that I do my best to live up to. Dorothea and Waltraud became some of my best friends.
>
> I enjoyed working in the South Africa women's group too, of course, and got to know lots of wonderful people, such as Rev. Leni Altwegg, the stalwart opponent of apartheid. Through the

group, I also got in touch with the South Africa Boycott Group, and got to know some more dedicated individuals, like Ursula Walter and Peter Gessler of the development policy organisation "Declaration of Berne," as well as Mascha Madörin, an expert on banking questions involving Switzerland and South Africa. Vreni Schneider was also involved behind the scenes. They all contributed to important information campaigns and direct actions against apartheid.

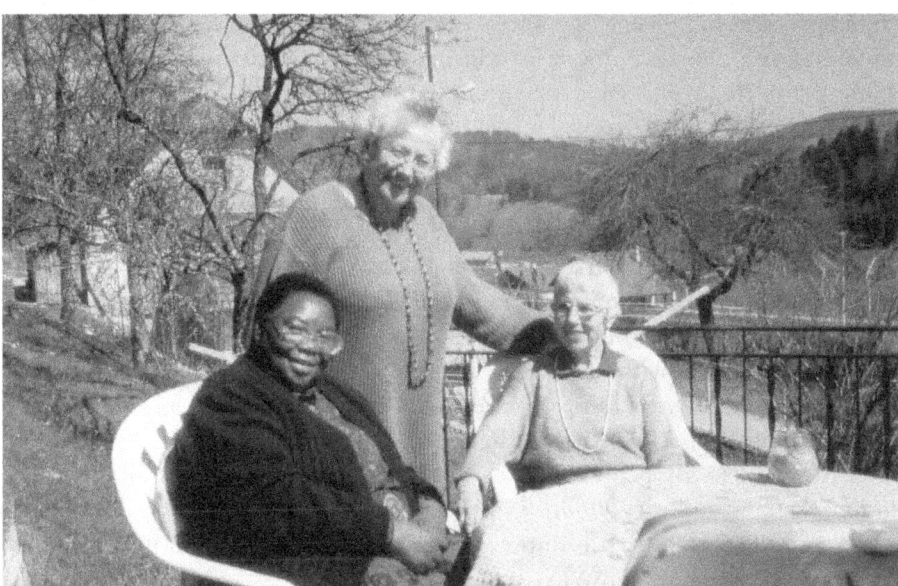

At Gertrud Stiehle's beloved home in the Jura: Selina, Gertrud and Dorothea Rüsch

Well-informed due to her connections with the anti-apartheid movement, Erika made an important personal decision in 1985: she closed her bank account with the *Schweizerische Kreditanstalt* (now Crédit Suisse). She made this decision because of the bank's support of the apartheid government, and wrote and told them why she was withdrawing her custom. The bank officials responded with a letter explaining that the South African Government was not as bad as people thought. This led to a long back-and-forth correspondence with the bank, in which Erika told them about her first-hand experience of what apartheid meant for black Africans in South Africa. She still smiles with satisfaction when she thinks about it: "I was able to give them a history lesson". In search of a new bank, at each one she visited she went in and asked for Krugerrand (South African gold coins). When the bank offered them to her, she politely left without further ado. But at the Co-op bank, the bank clerk said apologetically: "We don't trade in Krugerrand, because we don't do any business with South Africa." "Good", said Erika, "then I'll join you. Can I open an account?"

Passing on knowledge and experience

One of the people Erika met in the Mission House was Gertrud Stiehle, who recruited speakers for events in church congregations and for the general public. Gertrud organised a number of engagements for Erika, a competent and knowledgeable speaker, and she had requests for numerous events throughout Switzerland. It opened up a broad field of activity, leading to even more new connections. She described it with pleasure:

> I was warmly received everywhere I went. One nice engagement, one of the first, was in Illnau, where I had to preach in the church service. After the service, Lydia Bitzer, our former nanny, was waiting for me – and so were the parents of the famous flautist Peter Lukas Graf, whom I had got to know while on holiday in Ticino in 1946. In this way, I was able to resume old friendships.

> I once had to give a presentation about trachoma at a conference of the Ophthalmological Society, where I got to know the ophthalmologist Dr Josef Jeker from Basel. He had worked in Africa himself and already knew a little bit about me. A bit later, he was in the audience when I spoke about the Care Groups in the Don Bosco Church in Basel. Among other things, I talked about how important it is for members of a family to have personal face cloths to avoid spreading eye infections, and also about the significance of vegetable gardens for better nutrition. After my presentation, there was time for questions from the audience. Josef Jeker also raised his hand and made a comment, using a delightful play on words that only works in Swiss German. He said that the women's groups had progressed from the "Wäschblätz" (washcloth) to the "Gmüesblätz" (vegetable patch).
>
> A special memory of mine is a church service on the first Sunday of Advent in 1987, at St. Peter's Church in Basel, under Rev. Werner Schatz, where I preached the sermon. Following the good advice of Vreni Schneider, I chose the Massacre of the Innocents as the Bible text for my sermon and recalled the student uprising in Soweto. Rev. Schatz also asked me to participate in celebrating Holy Communion, not only helping to distribute the bread and wine, but speaking the prayers that are part of the liturgy leading up to the sharing of the bread and wine . I really had to prepare myself well for this service. My brother and my sister-in-law – who were very critical listeners – were among the worshippers, and they were very impressed by my sermon.

Engagements like these enabled Erika to pass on her rich knowledge as well as to show, based on her own example, how missionary service abroad can contribute to sustainable development and to helping people help themselves. Through such activities, Erika got to know new people and networks in Switzerland that became important to her. And she also learned a great deal herself, thanks to her wide-ranging reading and conversations with others.

Experiences with apartheid, seen from afar – and the beginning of change

Another important learning process for Erika was being able to look back on her experiences with apartheid. It was only when she was in Switzerland that she could thoroughly examine what had happened and how things were developing, above all thanks to her contact with members of the church-based anti-apartheid movement. Looking back, she concluded:

> Those living outside Africa were better informed, and formed more radical opinions of the situation. While I was living in South Africa I had become accustomed to the apartheid system, perforce, and to a certain extent I had come to terms with the situation. I wanted to do my job, and I hoped at least to build a few bridges between black and white. Thinking of the "whites" I knew there, I can't simply pass negative judgment on them all, for I knew a number of Afrikaners who looked after their black employees with decency and honesty. And, as I mentioned before, I was very impressed by the "white" opposition movement. What is more, and this must also be said, there was an astonishing amount of resistance literature in South Africa, although the publishers, especially the Ravan Press, the SACC (South African Council of Churches), and the Christian Institute were under the constant surveillance of the secret police.

The beginning of change

In the years following her retirement, Erika repeatedly returned to South Africa to visit, and she noted the beginnings of a change. Even in the final years of apartheid, some of her long time African colleagues began to interact with her much more freely, simply because she was no longer an employee of the state. Following the transition to democracy under Nelson Mandela, she was impressed by the discovery that an integrated seminar could be held as a matter of course in a Game Reserve Centre that had previously been reserved for Africans. A European South African told her how the change felt personally liberating: "I no longer have to feel guilty for being white." But the experience that left the greatest impression on Erika occurred during her last visit to South Africa in 1996. She had the chance to participate in a hearing of the Truth and Reconciliation Commission in Toyuhandowu, about fifty kilometres from Elim:

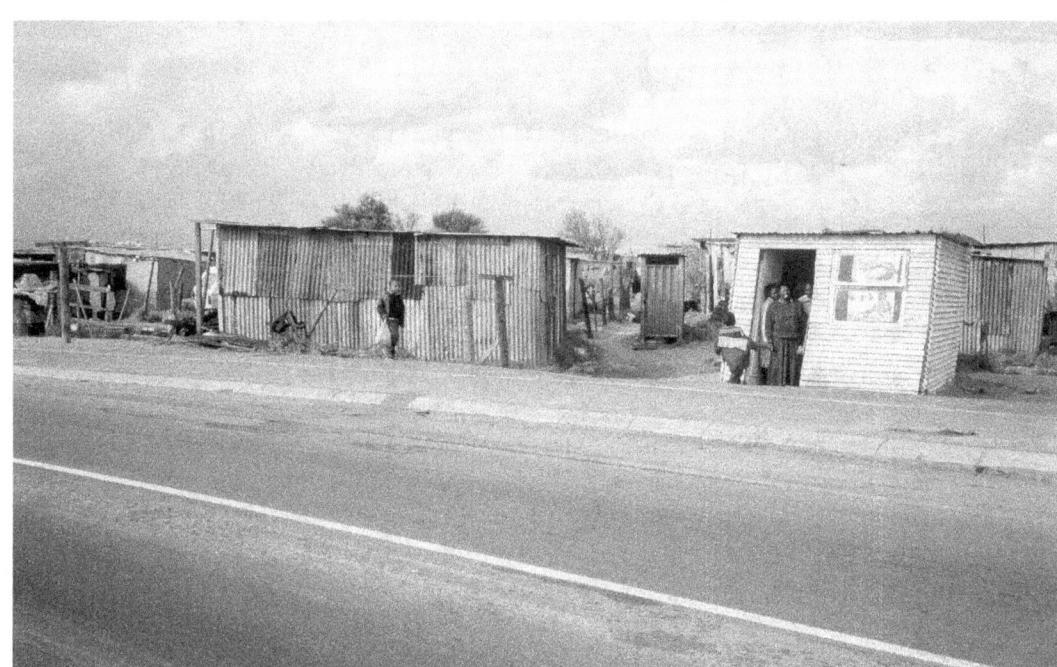

Khayelitsha, South Africa's second biggest township, 1996

It was terribly difficult to hear all these stories, so concentrated, one after another. I already knew a lot, and yet it made me physically ill – but I didn't want to leave the room because I knew they wouldn't let me back in. It was an extraordinary experience to see how people who had been tortured wanted to know exactly where and how this had happened. They had been kidnapped and abused, and they wanted to have clarity in order to forgive. I was deeply impressed by the Africans' capacity to forgive, provided they were told the truth about what had been done to them and by whom. It was moving to witness how nearly everyone was then truly able to forgive – a strength that we Europeans don't have. It was the mothers of those who had been tortured and murdered who couldn't forgive. It was very important for the victims to be able to publicly discuss what had been done to them. In some cases, they were even able to confront the perpetrators.

New horizons

Retirement also finally gave Erika time to consider educational travel – something that she had refrained from for many years. So, in 1985, she spontaneously agreed to join an old schoolmate on a study trip to China. Why not? Having skimped on vacations in Africa, she still had enough money saved up to pay for the expedition. However, when she got back she announced, "No more group tours for me!" as some of the participants had been very unpleasant. Nevertheless, she eventually let her brother Ernst and his wife Gaby persuade her to join them on a hiking and cultural tour of Egypt, which turned out to be beautiful, and inspires her to this day. The tour guide was very knowledgeable. He did not only show them the backdrop of ancient Egyptian tradition, but also pointed out how links between Jewish, Egyptian and Christian cultures had been influenced by Jewish and Christian traditions in that part of the world. She then had the pleasure of two lovely trips to Russia with Gaby, organised by Basel's Old Catholic *(Christkatholische)* Church, which enabled her to gain fascinating insights into the Russian Orthodox Church.

However, after so many years in Africa, Erika's biggest wish was to get to know Europe better and, above all, to rediscover Switzerland. Accustomed to the brown, yellow and grey colours of the African landscape, her eyes could not get enough of the lush green forests, hills, and fields. Until a few years ago, she was able to undertake extensive hiking, art, and music tours throughout Europe together with friends and family. Today, she limits herself to less distant journeys; for example, hotel vacations with a friend in her beloved Splügen, in the Hinterrhein area, or holidays for seniors with her friend Rev. Marianne Graf Grether.

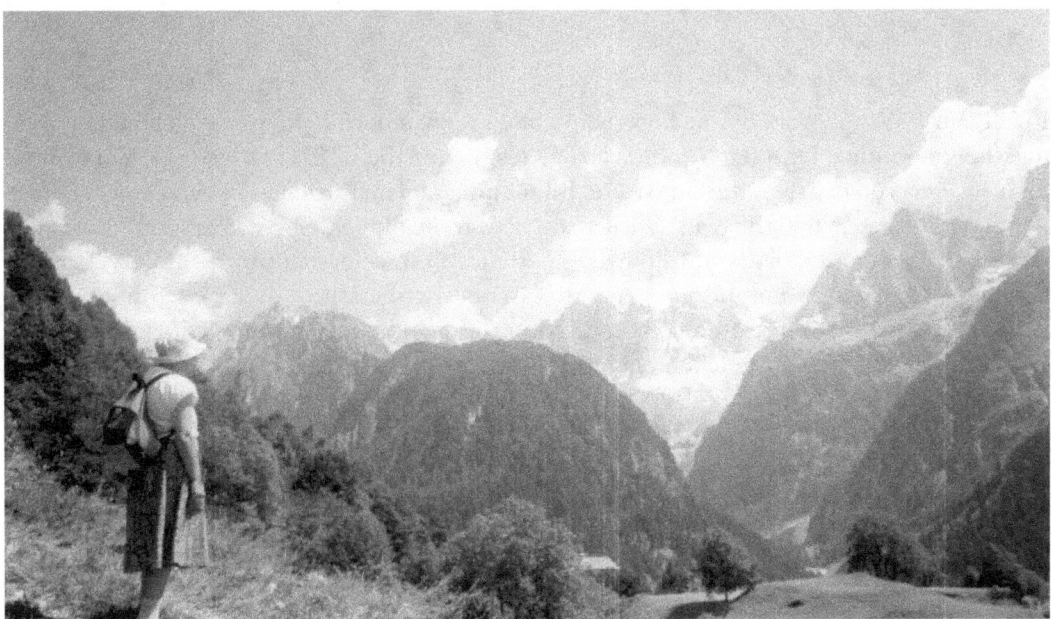

In Soglio, 1998

Teaching in London and in Basel – and books about the Care Groups

Retirement brought not only new opportunities for travel, but also new professional challenges. While she was still in South Africa, Erika had begun to look for something useful to do after retirement. In 1985 she began to teach both in England and in the Swiss Tropical Institute in Basel (now the Swiss Tropical and Public Health Institute) at practically the same time. She spent several years commuting regularly between London and Basel.

Teaching at the London International Centre for Eye Health (ICEH)

The teaching in England was at the International Centre for Eye Health (ICEH). As a result of the two presentations she had given at the international symposium she had attended in 1984, a few weeks before she retired, the ICEH asked her to teach a regular course on preventive village level eye care. She did this with pleasure for ten years. However, she wanted to do more than lecture – she wanted to pass on her knowledge in book form so it would reach a wider audience. At that time, there was only one book available on ophthalmology in developing countries, and that was only concerned with curative medicine, and contained nothing on prevention. Before she left Elim, Erika had put together an extensive handbook on preventive eye care in rural areas in the South, for the use of the teaching staff of the School for the Diploma in Ophthalmic Nursing. She showed this to the director of the ICEH, Professor Barry Jones, and convinced him of the need to make something of it. But she only wanted to undertake the work with a team, and finding a team proved difficult. However, Erika did not give up the idea of the book. This was one reason why she returned to Elim in 1986 to visit Selina:

> I told her in advance about the reason for my trip. I wanted to conduct interviews with her, because I absolutely had to learn more about the Care Groups as they really were. I realised that I had increasingly come to idealise them in my lectures and courses in Europe. I needed to come down to earth and learn again about the reality of life in the groups, and their problems. I needed to be able to depict things accurately, especially as I was still hoping that a book would eventually be feasible

Hanyane – a book about eye care for community health workers.

Finally, in 1987, the work on the book could begin. A wonderful group of collaborators came together in London. Dr Allen Foster, who had just joined the ICEH as a lecturer, had worked for many years on behalf of the Christoffel Blindenmission in Tanzania. Victoria Francis, from South Africa, also joined the team. That was a real stroke of luck. She was a talented communications expert and illustrator, who had experience in development work and was very interested in the issues around eye care. It turned out that she was also a friend of Erika's friend Frances Lund from Durban. Now they could get started! Erika showed the team the handbook that she had prepared as a teaching aid. Its basis was an everyday village story:

> The story centres on a mother whose child gets measles and goes blind. The mother receives no support from her husband, as is so often the case, since he left to go to Johannesburg in search of work and started another family there. The child is malnourished and suffers from severe vitamin A deficiency. Since a measles infection consumes lots of vitamin A, blindness often occurs within days. It's not a problem that can simply be solved in the hospital – you have to go after the causes.

> The editorial team decided to use this story framework as a narrative thread that would run through the whole book, accompanied by consistent illustrations of the characters and their environment to enable easier identification. Each episode of the story is followed by a discussion of related health issues, and a few questions for the reader to answer – for his or her own environment. The intention is to link theory with practice, which is something that is often not encouraged in schools in countries where resources are limited. The book's structure also invites readers to act out scenes from the story spontaneously – something that Africans are really good at!

The book was given the name *Hanyane: a village struggles for Eye Health*. It was intended as a primer for those involved in health work in rural areas. It was finally published in late 1989 in English by Macmillan, with financial help from the ICEH, the Royal National Society for the Blind (UK) and the *Christoffel Blindenmission*. It was eventually published in French, Hindi, and Bengali as well.

It was very exciting for Erika to know that the book had appeared. Early in the morning of January 2nd 1990, she received a telephone call from the Basel-Mulhouse airport. A 50 kilogram box had arrived for her! She knew it contained the free copies of *Hanyane* that she had been promised. She was still lying in bed as the telephone rang and when she tried to get up she had an unexpected shock. She suddenly realised that she could no longer control her left leg or her left hand! It was a mild stroke, and fortunately caused only temporary paralysis. Nothing too dramatic – but the signs of age were beginning to show!

Teaching at the Swiss Tropical Institute

Erika's teaching in the Swiss Tropical Institute in Basel, under its new Director, Professor Antoine Degrémont, began in 1985 – the same year as her teaching in London. For the next 14 years, she gave lectures on practising ophthalmology in the South in the Institute's courses on tropical medicine. Whenever there was space for it in her lectures, Erika discussed the Care Groups. However, the wider significance of this pioneer work in community health care, and what Erika had built up with the Care Groups, was first recognised in 1990 by the next Director of the STI, Professor Marcel Tanner, after he had read *Hanyane*.

At around this time, there was also less demand for the teaching of ophthalmology as part of the course in Tropical Medicine. The course had been reorganised, and the clinical part was no longer taught in Basel, but in Ifakara in Tanzania, where the STI has long-standing links to a hospital and research centre. The emphasis of the course in Basel, which was taught in English, was more on Health Management and Health Services, including community health. This change enabled Erika to focus her lectures exclusively on primary health care and trachoma.

The students were a diverse group. They came from different professions associated with health care; there were doctors, nurses, health care organisers and others – both women and men. About half of them were from Europe – mostly Swiss and Germans. Most of them already had experience of serving in a developing country, or hoped to work in one in the future. The others came from many different countries in Asia, Africa and South America. One thing they had in common was that they all had at least three years professional experience behind them.

Erika recalls:

> In most years, I was very well received by the students. On one occasion, the course participants independently put together a session about development that covered all the issues, including financial questions. Following my introductory lecture, one student made a presentation about the origins of development aid in general and Switzerland's role in particular. Switzerland's contributions to development were compared to the financial sums that Switzerland derived from developing countries. The latter were demonstrably higher than the funds flowing from Switzerland to the South. It was fascinating.

> However, it was not the same every year. The next class was the complete opposite. All the lecturers suffered, myself included. There were a number of disagreeable students from Germany who were used to sitting by while someone gave lectures, and who refused to participate actively. I didn't impress them at all. In their final evaluations, they said that the elderly lady clearly meant well in what she said, but that it was much too missionary for their taste.

One of the course leaders, Dr Felix Küchler, did his best to comfort Erika. He said the group had driven him to distraction too, and that she shouldn't take their evaluation seriously. But it bothered her all the same, especially since the previous course had gone so much better. And besides – being suddenly deemed irrelevant is unsettling.

These years also gave rise to a delightful new experience. In 1988, Selina Maphorogo went to Manchester for a course of study, and visited Erika on the way. An opportunity arose for Selina to describe the Care Groups and her work with them to the students and staff of the STI in a lunch break during Erika's course at the Tropical Institute. She described things in a very lively and practical way, and also talked about the difficulties. It was well received by everyone present. Professor Tanner and the staff of the Health Management Course were very impressed, and from 1996 to 1999 Selina was officially invited to contribute to the course together with Erika. The Tropical Institute funded her trips two or three times, but eventually decided that the cost was too high for a half-day course contribution.

A new book about the Care Groups

Professor Tanner was not only enthusiastic about the course on the Care Groups, but about Erika's plan for a new book, that would tell the story of Selina Maphorogo's work, and how the project developed. He helped with suggestions about funding organizations, and suggested that Jennifer Jenkins, an English scientist who was working in the Tropical Institute, should edit the book. The resulting book, *The Community is my University*, was finally published in 2003, and all the graduates of the Tropical Institute's course that year were given a copy as a parting gift.

Why did Erika want to publish yet another book? *Hanyane*, the textbook for primary health care practitioners, which had been published by Macmillan in 1989, was still available. But Erika felt it was very important that her colleague and close friend Selina Maphorogo should be given a voice – and not only her, but all the other "grassroots workers" as well. Selina is very good at articulating the problems encountered in her grassroots-level work, while others do not dare to do so for fear of losing their jobs. But she would never have written a book on her own. The writing of *The Community is my University* was a collaborative effort. Erika recorded and transcribed innumerable interviews with Selina. She and Jennifer Jenkins worked together to structure the mass of material so that it would tell Selina's story as vividly as it deserved. It is the story of the growth and development of the Care Groups as a grassroots movement, including all the successes and frustrations. The book portrays the transformation of Selina's role from that of Erika's assistant to that of the leader of a community movement. Erika's own contribution to the book describes the background of the Care Groups and the need for a community approach to health, while the epilogue, written together with Erika's successor Carel IJsselmuiden and her colleague Peter Kok expands the focus to encompass a global perspective.

Honours

Over the years, Erika Sutter has received numerous awards to honour her life's work in the prevention of blindness and the promotion of community health care and development. Whenever possible at an awards ceremony, Erika points out that she did not earn a particular honour on her own, but rather in collaboration with her team partner Selina Maphorogo.

First among the honours she received was "Woman of the Year" in South Africa. Just months after her arrival back in Switzerland, Erika was invited by the liberal South African daily newspaper The Star to come to South Africa for the concluding event at which the Woman of the Year, as chosen by readers, would be announced. To her great surprise, she was chosen out of many candidates and awarded the prize in front of television cameras. She also recalls that:

A journalist from the state-owned South African radio station interviewed me and asked, "What will you tell them in Switzerland about South Africa?" I responded, "The truth." His jaw literally dropped – and my response was never broadcast.

This particular visit to South Africa also gave Erika a chance to catch up with her Care Group successor, Dr Carel IJsselmuiden, in Elim. He had accumulated six months of experience with the Care Groups in the meantime, and the meeting gave them a chance to discuss questions that had come up for him. Erika had the pleasure of seeing that "her" project was progressing well.

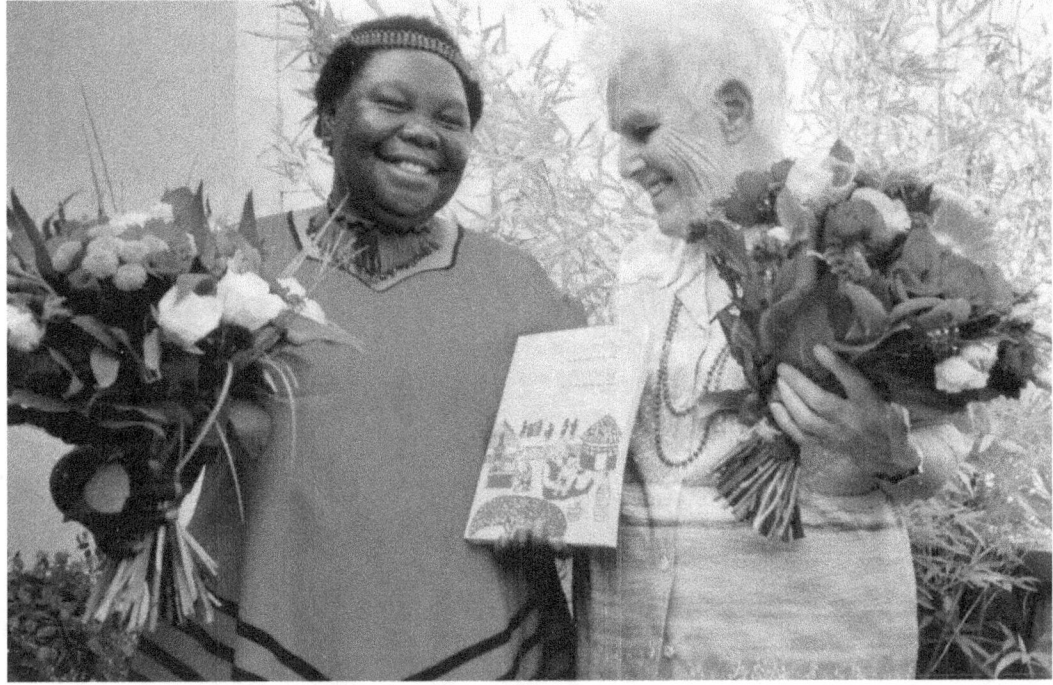

Selina and Erika are awarded Honorary Diplomas by the STI in 2004

In 1995, the University of Basel's Faculty of Medicine nominated Erika for an honorary doctorate. The Dean of the Faculty, Prof. Josef Flammer, Professor of Ophthalmology, presented her with the certificate.

Just one year later, the French *Ligue Internationale contre le Trachome* awarded her the Trachoma Gold Medal and invited her to Paris for the ceremony. This turned out to be a real adventure. The award included a gold medal and a cash prize. This time, Erika succeeded in persuading the prize committee to divide the award between herself and her South African partner. Erika was set to receive the medal, while Selina would receive the cash prize. The two arranged their train trip to Paris, and finally arrived at a huge conference building, where nobody at the reception desk had ever heard of the *Ligue Internationale contre le Trachome*. Eventually, they found the right room, after a long odyssey through the building – and the organisers were cross with them because they were late. After the meeting they were simply left standing, and not offered any hospitality, or any compensation for their travel or other expenses. However, they enjoyed Paris nevertheless. The brother of Erika's friend Marie-Claire Barth in Basel offered them a place to stay, and they enjoyed a couple of days touring the wonderful city and being together. As they strolled through the city, Selina proved to be a great tour guide with her hawk eyes and her excellent sense of direction, so Erika, with her poor eyesight, could entrust everything to her.

Erika is especially pleased about an honour given to her in 2005, 20 years after she had left South Africa, by the Ophthalmological Society of South Africa, in recognition of her humanitarian engagement. She would never even have known about it had it not been for a Swiss ophthalmologist working in Bloemfontein, whom she had never met before. He called her after the event, when he came to Switzerland for a short leave, and then personally delivered the certificate on behalf of the South African organization. It gives her a great sense of satisfaction to know that people still knew her name in South Africa twenty years after her departure, and she sees it as a sign of the sustainability of her work, both in the Care Groups and in preventive eye care.

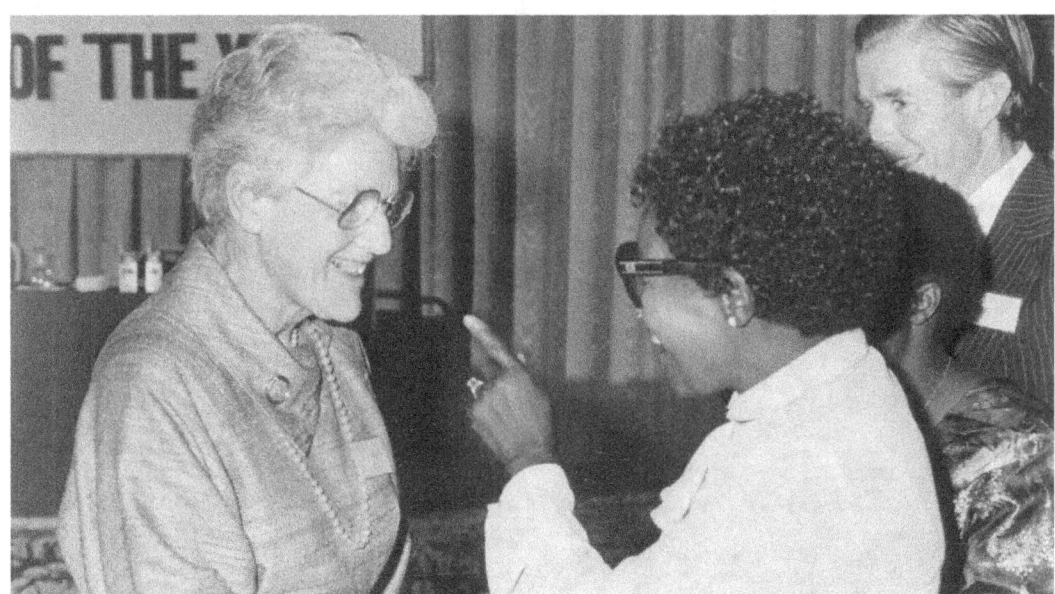

Erika is honoured as "Woman of the year" by the South African liberal newspaper The Star, 1984

Drawing strength from family

What keeps Erika feeling firmly grounded during the many, often very challenging, experiences and activities she pursues in her retirement? Besides faith and good friendships, it is above all Erika's family; a family in which she – single, and with no children of her own – is warmly embedded. Everyone loves her. One of her older brother Hans's three daughters in Lausanne, Brigitte, Erika's goddaughter, always has a guest bed ready for her when she comes to Lausanne for meetings with the *Département Missionnaire*. The two really appreciate one another and regularly get in touch. Erika's relationship with her brother Ernst, his wife Gaby, and their four children was always near and dear. While Ernst was alive, they often went on holiday together in their house in Berzona in Ticino, or undertook other pleasant trips. Today, Erika and Gaby regularly meet for meals, to play Scrabble, or to enjoy the monthly Bach cantatas at the Old Catholic *(Christkatholische)* church. Erika knows she can count on her sister-in-law in any emergency. To her delight, she also has an excellent relationship with her niece and three nephews from this family, all of whom live in Basel. Of course, they all have jobs and are kept quite busy, but Erika accepts that the members of the younger generation are usually pressed for time. When she feels it is too long since they heard from each other she gets in touch with a telephone call. And the fact that time spent together is rare makes it all the more precious.

One person is especially dear to Erika: Christian, her godson, the son of her brother Ernst. From a very young age, he showed a great affection for his *Gotte* (godmother) Erika, whom he called "Riggi", whenever she came from faraway Africa to visit Basel. She recalls:

> When Christian was five, around the start of my medical studies, I came to Switzerland and spent a winter holiday with him in Davos. We went on a ride in a horse-drawn sleigh, and I can still picture his reaction to this day: completely quiet, simply overcome with awe. On another day, we had to cross a street that had an icy patch. He looked up at me and said: "I'll give you my hand so you won't fall!"
>
> Once, while I was in Africa, I painted him a picture book, based on the story of "Mamabo", a black girl in an African fairytale song. Later on, once when he was really sick, I drew a kiss from Mamabo on a letter I sent him. She became so real in his imagination that he asked on my next visit, "Why didn't you bring Mamabo?" So I gave him a Tsonga rag doll with the same name, which he has to this day.

During Erika's training period at the Basel Eye Hospital, Christian, now twelve years old, was occasionally allowed to visit his godmother at the hospital:

> I showed him the doctors' room with all its facilities. He was especially attracted to the dictaphone, and then he wanted to test his vision, of course. Two months later, a new test showed that Christian had become near-sighted. This can occur very quickly during preadolescence. So we were able to outfit him with the correct spectacles right away. In addition, he always had a striking number of bruises, and almost bled to death from a tonsillectomy. It turned out he had haemophilia. Luckily, the diagnosis was made just before a necessary appendectomy. Last of all, he began complaining about hip problems, which I investigated. His parents and I might have been tempted to think that he was coming up with illnesses simply because his godmother was visiting from Africa – but sure enough, he was in the early stages of a hip disease. Fortunately it could be treated without surgery, by avoiding stress on the hip joints. So, fresh out of university, I was able to put my general medical knowledge to good use for my godson.

Erika and Christian regularly wrote letters to each other, in which Erika became something of a confidant for him during adolescence. Later, when he insisted that he didn't want to complete the high school course, ending with the Matura examination, but rather wished to go straight to the Conservatorium to train as a double-bass player, his parents asked Erika to have a serious word with him. But it didn't do any good. He remained determined. His parents eventually gave up and agreed to finance his music studies, and he graduated with flying colours from the Music Academy in Basel. As a professional musician, he has stayed true to the double bass to this day, and he has also stayed true to his "Gotte Riggi", who continues to listen keenly to his concerts. On her eightieth birthday, he delighted her by telling the story of Mamabo, accompanied by his double bass.

Limited time, and thoughts of death

On her eightieth birthday, Erika sensed very strongly for the first time: "From now on, my lifetime is limited." Her remaining time grows ever more precious – her "time-yet," as her friend Margrith refers to it. It is good to reconcile the past and come to terms with things, enabling the discovery of new meaning, and unfettered appreciation of the remaining time one is given. Erika's friend Rev. Marianne Graf has offered her pastoral guidance in these years, for which she is very grateful.

Naturally, Erika's thoughts also revolve around death at times. She has experienced it often: in her family, in Africa and in other cultures, and would like to learn to accept it in her own life. Her memories return to the year 1945, when she lost sister Trudi and her father within three months of one another:

Erika's nephew and godson Christian at her 90th birthday party, 2007

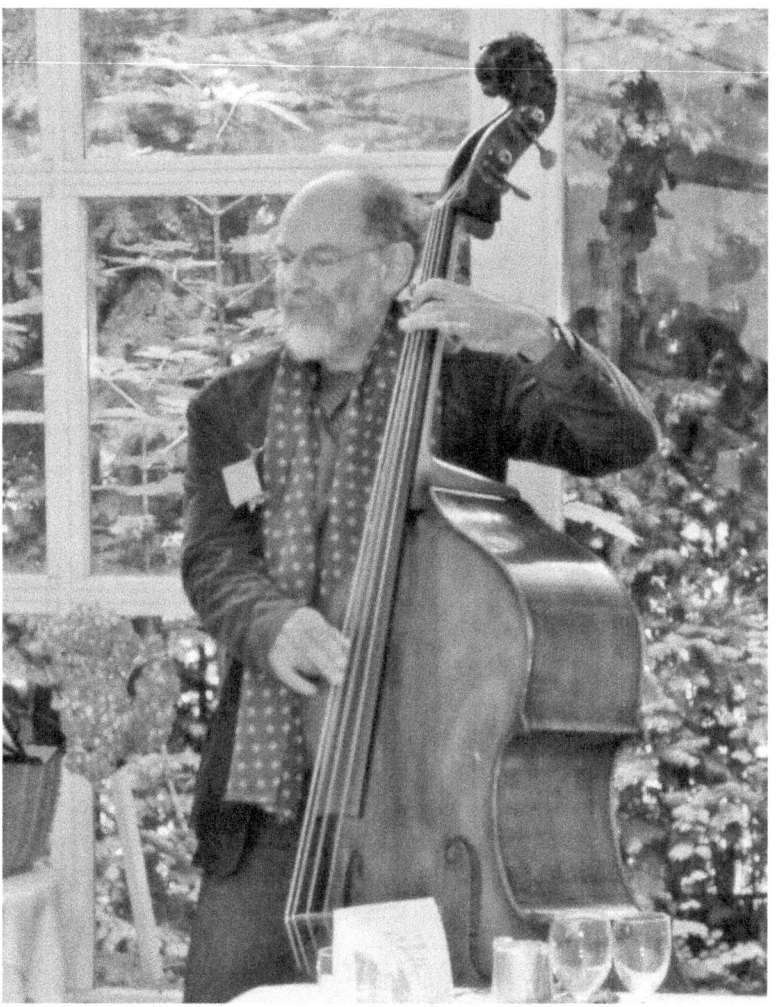

I had a close relationship with my sister Trudi, who was eight years older. She was very dear to me. She was ill for a long time. We shared her final night – the hours of crisis. I think she enjoyed listening to me play my viola da gamba. She seemed a bit better in the morning, so I was able to go to work at Roche. About eleven o'clock my mother called, "Come quickly!" Trudi regained consciousness one final time, as if she had waited for me. I recited the Lord's Prayer with her, and during the appeal "forgive us our trespasses", she passed away.

Trudi, the fighter, had finally laid down her life. Yet she remained palpably present for Erika for many years. And, as if it happened of its own accord, Erika steadily took on Trudi's role in the years that followed, gradually developing a fighting spirit that she had never needed while under Trudi's wing. But Erika takes pains to clarify that, in contrast to Trudi, she didn't dare openly to display that fighting spirit.

Shortly after Trudi's death, Erika's father died at home from the complications of a stroke. At the end, he was no longer able to speak, which was very sad for everyone around him. He finally died alone – of all things, on the very night when Erika had been able to persuade her mother to go to the opera Fidelio with her! That was very difficult for her mother to bear.

Erika's mother died later, when Erika was in South Africa, and was unable to be there and to say goodbye. At the hour of her mother's death on Advent Sunday in 1962, Erika was playing the viola da gamba in Johannesburg's Lutheran Church, and she only learned the bad news afterwards in letters from her aunt and her brother Ernst. It came as a great shock. Why did her mother have to die precisely at a time when she was having difficulty responding to her regular letters to Africa? And after a lifetime of difficulty between them? Now there would be no chance to be reconciled with one another. These feelings led to a depression. Luckily, a little later, Erika received a lovely letter from Rev. Marianne Kappeler, in which she described her mother's final days and her love for Erika, which Erika had rarely felt during her lifetime. It was only many years later that Erika was able to mourn for her mother and feel she understood her better.

Like Trudi, Ernst continued to be very present in Erika's life following his death in November 1999. He often appeared in her dreams, always as someone there to help her in a difficult situation. She still misses her trusted childhood playmate, whose pursuits as a scientist, ornithologist and rose-lover further endeared him to her. Just before his death, he wanted to give her roses for her eighty-second birthday – the plants remain on her balcony as his legacy, continuing to bloom year after year. When he lay dying in the St. Clara Hospital, fully aware of his condition, Erika visited him every day. She respected his views as an agnostic, but was able to read and discuss with him a text by Dietrich Bonhoeffer about the fragmentariness of life. The very last text that Ernst was able to read was Akhenaten's "Hymn to Aten (the Sun Goddess)." He read aloud to Erika his favourite lines:

> Hark to the chick in the egg,
> he who speaks in the shell!
> You give him air within
> to save and prosper him;
> And you have allotted to him his set time
> before the shell shall be broken;
> Then out from the egg he comes,
> from the egg to peep at his natal hour!
> And up on his own two feet goes he
> when at last he struts forth therefrom.[1]

The importance of saying goodbye and grieving is something that Erika has witnessed time and again in other cultures:

> During a trip to Russia with Gaby, we visited a Russian Orthodox church. It had three aisles. A baptism was taking place on the left side, in the middle a wedding was underway, and a funeral was being held on the right side. According to Orthodox custom, the deceased is laid out for three days in an open coffin in the church. During that time, one can view the body and say "Goodbye". Afterwards is the burial, at which the deceased's family personally nails the coffin shut. It strikes me as a very beautiful part of the grieving process, enabling one to participate in a physical act of saying goodbye, not solely a spiritual one. That way one can grasp it. This is how it is now.

> I witnessed other examples of death rites in Africa. When my laboratory assistant Julius died, I delivered the news to his family in a remote village. The villagers immediately began wailing and lamenting. This is a necessary act that belongs to the death rites of many cultures. Once I went with Selina to visit the widow of someone who had just died. After we had sat with her for a while, a group of youths came along and sang, then another person came and prayed, and so on. Selina explained that someone was always with the deceased's family in the time between the death and the burial, day and night. They were never left alone. I think that's very beautiful.

Erika with her brother Ernst at his bird exhibition at the Natural History Museum in Basel, 1989

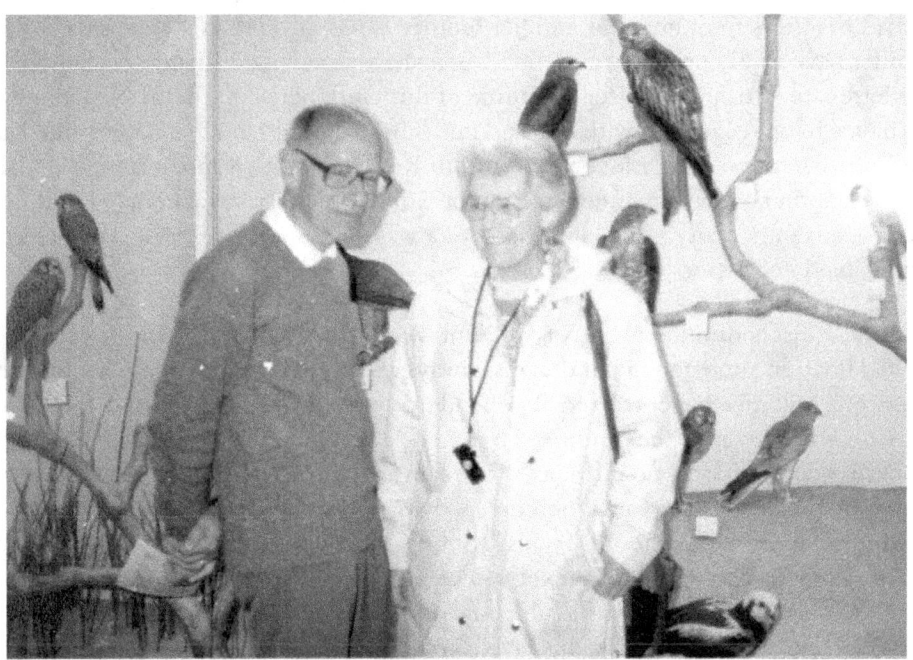

The death of her friend Irène Bourcart in 2005 triggered a decisive realisation in Erika that one must make preparations in good time. It happened like this:

> I was on vacation with my sister-in-law at her home in Ticino, when we received a phone call informing us of Irène's death. I travelled back to Basel for the funeral, of course, promising Gaby I would confirm my arrival after the long train ride. But there were complications during the trip, so I wasn't able to call until late at night, and she didn't hear the telephone. She was really worried about me, and said: "You know, if something had happened to you, we wouldn't have known how to organise everything according to what you wanted." After that, the two of us put together a list of all my instructions, which I adjust as necessary every once in a while.

Now things are in order. Erika continues to enjoy life and is glad to have made all the preparations. Yet there are dark moments too:

> When it comes down to it, I don't know how I'll react. Sometimes, when I feel ill at night and the fear of death catches me, I think to myself that I don't want to die yet, that there's still so much that I have to do and arrange. I don't bother with thinking about the hereafter. It will certainly be very different from what all theories or desires say it will be. It is much more the actual moment of dying that frightens me. But I hope that it will be the same for me as it has been for many others, and that when the time comes I will want to die.

Endnote

1 Translated by John L. Foster, published in: *Ancient Egyptian Literature: An Anthology*, University of Texas Press, Austin, 2001.

IX A final look back and forward

A conversation between Erika Sutter (E) and Gertrud Stiehle (G)

After the long collaborative journey leading to the creation of this biography, it seems both appropriate and important to add a final chapter of reflection, tying together the key experiences of Erika Sutter's life from her own perspective, and venturing a look ahead at the final phase. The following *"tour d'horizon"* – in the form of direct conversation between Erika Sutter (E) and Gertrud Stiehle (G) – helps to reveal the inner logic of Erika's rich life, one in which detours and setbacks have ultimately led to a sense of fulfilment and gratitude.

We would also like to take this opportunity to extend special thanks to Frances Lund, whose brilliant idea and constant support made this book possible.

G: Dearest Erika, your memories and your life have finally been committed to paper, and will be accessible to many people, including readers in countries of the global South, which is very important to you. What has the whole process meant to you?

E: This biography came about thanks to the encouragement of a friend in South Africa, Frances Lund, who was very familiar with my life's work. "Another book?" I found myself asking sceptically. "Perhaps for the sake of the Care Group members, who might want to know a little bit about me... But who else would be interested in my life?"

It was clear from the beginning that I couldn't write an autobiography on my own, and that, at most, I could tell the story of my life to someone – a person whom I trusted, and one who I was confident would articulate things well, and make something good out of it. That person is you. You helped me get my memories flowing and, with that, set the whole process in motion. I jumped from one memory to the next, no doubt chaotically at times, but that's just how it is. That's also how my life's course initially appeared to me – zig-zagging this way and that; fragmented in some places – until I began the biography work with you. From then on, I began to pick up on the continuity in my life and the connections between things. It's a good way of processing the past. Indeed, it's been good for me.

G: But wasn't it stressful for you? I've demanded a lot of you at your advanced age.

E: Oh, yes. I often felt I was reaching my limit, and possibly I could have used more breaks, but because you kept pushing, I kept going. I also want to be there to see this book published, being ninety-four already! I allowed myself more time on my previous two books, but sensed even then that it came at the expense of social contact. Afterwards, for instance, I scarcely had any energy to invite friends over, and nowadays it's even harder to make up for this. Since then, some of my dear old friends have passed away and others simply aren't up to joint activities anymore. Some things are irretrievably gone.

G: You and I, we had two very different perspectives on your life, as seen from the outside and from the inside. Did that also become apparent to you?

E: These changes of perspective introduced some useful suspense into our joint adventure. I often had the feeling that you see me as a much better person than I think I am. But I've often felt that way with others, too. Perhaps that is why I love the poem by Dietrich Bonhoeffer: "Who am I?" *(Wer bin ich?)*. In it, he asks himself who he is, how others see him, and ends by saying: "Whoever I am – I'm yours, oh Lord."

G: You mentioned seeing connections in your life now. Is there a common thread running through it that ties things together?

E: Yes, I would say so. The *cantus firmus*, from the realm of music, would be an apt metaphor – the melody that flows through an entire piece of music. In the case of Bonhoeffer, who I've often looked to over the years, it is God who brings together the fragments of human life and creates a whole. In my case, it's thanks to you that I've discovered the existence of a continuous path weaving its way through my life.

G: Let's take a look at some recurrent themes in your life. You said once that you had three career choices: the natural sciences, social work, and theology – what happened with them?

E: All three of them eventually played an important part in my life, especially during my time in South Africa, in which I was everything; scientist, doctor, missionary, and social worker.

G: Let's stay with the natural sciences for a moment. Would you say there's a direct line connecting the little girl who didn't want to step on any Alpine flowers to the elderly woman who today enjoys spending time on her balcony garden, keeps up with environmental issues, and is concerned about our planet's survival?

E: Yes. In Africa I first worked as a biologist in charge of the hospital laboratory, and then, after my medical studies, I invested myself body and soul in my work as an ophthalmologist. In later years, aspects of social engagement came more to the fore in my work on behalf of community health care. But when I had a little time off, I enjoyed observing all the animals in the national parks. Once I went in the company of my brother Ernst, when he came to attend an All-Africa Ornithological Congress that I had told him about. Back in Switzerland, I've rediscovered the Alpine flora and the joy of identifying plants on many hiking trips with my friend Margrith. For my eightieth birthday, my family gave me the botanical "bible" *Flora Helvetica,* which is very precious to me. Seventy years ago, there were already clues pointing to the environmental problem of over-fertilised lakes (for example, the lakes of Hallwil and Sempach).

When I returned to Switzerland in 1984, our ailing forests and the threat of climate change were the main focuses of those concerned about the environment. Those people were considered somewhat eccentric at the time, but since then these problems have acquired real urgency. For my own part, I consider it my responsibility to do everything I can so that my nephews and nieces and their descendants may have a future. I separate my rubbish for recycling, reuse plastics as much as possible, save water – especially hot water – and buy organic produce directly from the producers whenever possible, so as to strengthen organic farming. My friend Dorothea has been a real role model for me in such things, because of her steadfast dedication.

It's a constant source of concern for me how our drive for progress and money causes problems that our politicians are seldom willing to address. I continue to sign petitions to protect the environment, of course; I read a lot; and I'm a member of the organization International Physicians for the Prevention of Nuclear War. I suppose there's a reason my nieces and nephews refer to me as "the well-informed auntie"!

G: Now let's consider your commitment to social issues, which already began when you were a schoolgirl.

E: In Africa, I further developed my social engagement side mainly in my work with the Care Groups. As an ophthalmologist, I could never be indifferent to the question of why there was so much illness among the blacks in Africa. The South African Council for the Blind, and some care-givers in Elim, attributed the Africans' higher rate of blindness – in comparison with Europeans in South Africa and people in the West – to indigenous ignorance. I told myself that didn't make sense. The main problem is poverty. Don't Africans show an enormous amount of imagination, creativity, and courage just to carve out an existence with the most meagre of resources? My commitment to greater justice and human dignity has practical consequences. It isn't irrelevant to me where I buy my T-shirts. Supporting fair trade – equitable, sustainable methods of production and commerce – even when it costs more, means a little less poverty and injustice. I recall with pleasure the European Ecumenical Assembly entitled Peace, Justice and the Integrity of Creation, which was held in Basel in 1989. In an exhibition that was part of the event, many small groups of young people presented alternative projects and initiatives. That sort of thing continues to give me hope, even when nowadays the writings of someone like Jean Ziegler[1] make plain the hard facts and statistics of growing poverty and violence, which could lead one to doubt. One just has to live with this tension!

G: Behind the statistics, of course, there are always people. There's a Tsonga proverb that means a lot to you: "People are a goldmine". Why?

E.: I think it works on two levels that have been important to me in life: my belief that everyone has golden abilities, and my experience that people themselves have shaped and enriched my life like golden treasures.

G: There would be yet another level of interpretation – the exploitation of people like a goldmine! But you certainly don't mean that.

E: Of course not! During a visit to Gazankulu after my retirement in the late 1980s, I was very happy when the Care Groups were introduced at a workshop on development and someone remarked: "This was all made possible because someone believed in people!" That was and remains a central concern of mine. The South African Council for the Blind had a different attitude. They felt a project like the Care Groups wouldn't work out, claiming that the Africans couldn't think far enough ahead. They simply underestimated people. If anyone ever did appear to be less capable, it was mainly because of the dearth of educational opportunities and general lack of prospects, which, thankfully, is different nowadays. At the very beginning of my time in Africa, I also misjudged what people were capable of. My "lesson" took the form of my gifted laboratory assistant Julius, about whom others had said, "A black person can't do that!" When I got started with the Care Groups, I still thought you had to tell people just what they needed to do, until I learned that the opposite was true – thanks to Selina!

G: How did the missions view social work in the areas where they were working at that time?

E: For a long time it was a pretty one-sided "helper approach", giving people what they appeared to need. It was basically a donor and charity-recipient mentality, which strips the needy of their dignity and keeps them subordinate. At a conference of the Christoffel Blindenmission[2] in 1982, the motto was, "Bear one another's burdens". This was expounded as if to say that we, the strong ones, must bear the burdens of the weak, without seeing that they are perfectly capable of bearing their own burdens.

G: Social relations are a mutual give and take. During your life, what have you been given by others?

E: There have been many turning points in my life in which people have given me golden advice, supported me in my decisions, and been role models for me. Marie-Louise Martin, for example, first inspired me to pursue missionary service, and the Swedish medical missionary Dr Ysander gave me the decisive push. In 1949, he had written a small booklet called *The Bad Samaritan* which was very significant for me. In it, he states that Western medicine is not adequate for developing countries in Africa, and that it is better to reach people there by means of community health care. Work with people, not for them – that was his motto, which really made sense to me. Later on, Selina gave me very similar advice. For instance, she would say, "You must not blame the people" for their illness or for their use of harmful traditional practices. And she only practised constructive criticism that didn't diminish the person she was speaking with. For example, if she came across a mother who was shovelling maize porridge into her baby's mouth until it choked, coughed, and spluttered – to the point where it could get pneumonia – Selina didn't automatically scold her, but rather began by praising her. It is good, she would say, that you are giving your baby something healthy to eat, and it's also good to see that you wash your hands first. Only then would she offer advice: "Perhaps you can watch out that your baby doesn't gag at all, or else it might come down with pneumonia." She was always very sensitive about "victim-blaming".

Of course, I was also greatly enriched by my encounters with Beyers Naudé and my friendship with the African pastor Rev. Mpfumu in Elim.

G: And now for the third key thread running through your life, theology. What has been the course of your journey of faith?

E: It's been a lifelong up and down. My parental home wasn't especially influenced by Christianity. But even though my father was an agnostic, he considered it important for us to receive religious instruction and, equipped with our knowledge of Christianity, to make our own decisions later. My confirmation classes, conversations with Trudi, and active engagement in church youth work were important catalysts. The fact that I became a missionary doctor did not so much stem from a deep religious experience – though I did pray to make the right decision – as from a desire to practise a profession in a part of the world where I was really needed. It was a very workaday decision, quite free of romanticism.

In terms of my faith, my time in Africa was a bit of a drought. In our mission community, personal faith was a matter of course that wasn't questioned, and for me it felt rather paralysing. I recall few evangelicals who said anything inspiring; a secretary in Elim Hospital, maybe, or one of the members of the Student Christian Movement (SCM) which I joined during my medical studies in Johannesburg. But I never understood how some of the SCM members could make pastoral bedside visits to hospital patients they didn't know at all, and say pious things – often in English, which the unfortunate patient probably didn't even understand. Sometimes, during a furlough in Switzerland, I would have a chance to have a good theological discussion with Rev. Thurneysen in Basel, which helped me to "fill up my tank" a little. After my father died, my mother became almost fanatically religious and began writing down the sermons of Rev. Marianne Kappeler and sending them to me in Africa, which often felt like a burden to me. For my mother, this was an important step towards finding herself, towards the discovery of new interests and a sense of freedom, and I comforted myself with the thought that if this could happen to her so late in life, maybe there was still a chance that I too would find my way to a deeper sense of faith.

When I finally returned from Africa, my faith was pretty shallow, but I joined the organizing team of the women's group in my local church, St Stephen's, and simply participated, even though I felt that everyone else was much further in their faith than I was. This sort of continual practice appears to be a good way of overcoming dry spells. Fulbert Steffensky once said: "The lips are often wiser than the heart." When I got to know Waltraud Haas in the South Africa group, she gave me Kurt Marti's book *O Gott!* ("Oh God!") as a gift. Here, at last, was someone writing about things I felt were relevant – God here and now! Here was an anti-nuclear activist and a person concerned about the environment, whose religious and political language answered my needs. It was the same with the writings of Dorothee Sölle. Yes, that's the kind of faith I can practice. It is my great hope and wish that one day I may confidently give back the life that I have been given on trust.

G: But isn't there yet another, fourth thread running through your life – music?

E: Oh, yes. There was always lots of music in our family home. Of course, the driving force was my sister Trudi, the budding professional musician. She worked with me in particular. At the age of six or seven, I still couldn't really sing and had trouble with rhythm. I couldn't keep time, they said. We were always singing – while hiking, on vacation, or while washing dishes in the kitchen. I was given piano lessons for a little while, but I didn't enjoy them at all, especially not the teacher. However, when I was eleven, I decided to learn how to play the cello. Soon we were playing as a trio at home: Trudi on the violin, myself on the cello, and Mama on the piano (but she played too slowly). From then on, I grew up with the cello, which became my constant companion – on trips, in Sweden, and in Africa. I loved the instrument's deep, soft tones. When I gave it away a few years ago, I realised how much it had become a part of me. It was really painful when I had to stop playing because of my eyesight.

Musically, the richest years for me started in 1937, when Trudi began her studies of early music at the Schola Cantorum Basiliensis, which had been founded two years before. She was the school's first diploma student. I was also enthralled with early music. I took lessons on the recorder, sang in a choir with Ina Lohr, and – most importantly – took lessons on the bass viola da gamba with August Wenzinger. From then on, the bass viol was my favourite instrument. In the meantime, I had started my biology studies, and my parents thought, "She already has a cello, why does she need a viola da gamba as well?" So I had to earn the instrument. Despite my tough workload, I did all the shopping for the family, and was allowed to keep the stamps that were given to customers with each purchase and could eventually be exchanged for a cash bonus. That gave me enough for the special viol bow, and by tutoring I earned enough for the instrument itself.

G: What makes the viola da gamba so special? From a distance, it doesn't look very different from a cello, does it?

E: It has to do with particular qualities of the design, which lend many overtones to the resonance. As a result, the deep tones of the viola da gamba have an especially soft, high, singing sound.

G: Aren't you especially fond of your godson Christian Sutter, who, in his career as a passionate musician, opted for an instrument a size up from yours – the double bass?

E: Yes, I'm extremely proud of him. He also had to fight for the chance to study his instrument, and he's now an established, highly sought-after double bass player.

G: How did your interest in politics develop?

E: Early on, I was probably sensitised by my father, who was concerned about politics, and joined the Swiss *Freiwirtschafts-Bewegung* (movement for a free economy) of the late 1930s. During the Nazi period, we had many critical political discussions in my parental home, and because we took in Jewish refugees, we were very well informed about what was going on. Later on, in South Africa, it was impossible not to take a stance – at least in one's own mind – against apartheid. I didn't speak out openly, but I did try quietly to act against the apartheid regime. Beyers Naudé, who had fought against apartheid as a Christian, opened my eyes to a lot and showed me that you can't separate faith from politics. This became a guiding principle in my life. Once, during a workshop for Swiss missionaries in the 1980s, I made the statement: "If you are a Christian and a doctor, it is a 'must' to take an interest in politics", which greatly astonished some of the participants.

G: Now a totally different question: You've remained single all your life. Have you had any kind of surrogate family?

E: I never considered it anything special to live alone, and I also didn't have any difficulties later on in Elim. The Africans readily accept single white women, though for African women, being without husbands and children is still often a reason for discrimination.

For me, living alone means having a special sort of freedom – you can seek out and cultivate other forms of family. First of all, I'm very close to my extended family of nieces and nephews. What's more, the Care Groups are my family. Once, during one of my later visits, the members of a group gave me a Tsonga doll as a symbol of my "thousands of children". A few years ago, Selina called me on Mother's Day to congratulate me on being a mother to thousands of children. According to African tradition, of course, she and all her relatives and friends are my family too, and, vice versa, my relatives are considered hers. When she built her own house a few years ago, she included a room for me to use as I got older, so I would always have a place to stay. And her youngest son, Emmanuel, always signs his letters to me "Your loving son Emmanuel." When he was still really little, and could scream his lungs out, his siblings would plead, "Take him back to Doctor Sutter!" as they were convinced he was my son. I financed Emmanuel's training to become an expert horticulturalist, and have followed his career – working to beautify cities with parks and gardens – over the years. That has led to a special connection between us, of course.

And then there's little Selina – named after the grown-up one – who lives near Basel. She is the daughter of a Swiss couple, Sonja Horber and Markus Dörig, who spent a month in Elim in 1995, looking into the possibility of working for the Christoffel Blindenmission. They met Selina, and she became a close friend of theirs – so when their first daughter was born, shortly after their visit, they called her "Selina". Since then, the Dörigs have also become family to me; I am a grandmother to their children, Selina and Flurin, and have been deeply moved by the entire family's friendship and supportiveness.

When thinking about the topic of surrogate families, my circle of friends also comes to mind, of course, and especially the "missionary family." Brought together by chance, but sharing similar motivations for service in Africa, we mission workers have developed a strong bond that has held up over many years. Whenever possible, I go to the twice-yearly meetings, even though the older generation has shrunk considerably and there are scarcely any new members. Also at the central office of the *Département Missionnaire*, the few remaining staff members who know me and my projects are all close to retirement. This will lead, I sense, to a loss of continuity. The infusion of new ideas is a good thing, but it must build on the past. Older missionaries are often criticised today, as if they did everything wrong. They certainly made some mistakes too, but most of them were ahead of their time. The closeness experienced by my generation of mission workers is also crumbling for other reasons. Lifelong mission service no longer exists, and limited contracts and short missions have become the norm. This comes at the expense of really getting to know the local situation and people, which I think is a pity.

G: Getting older also means letting go. How has that been for you?

E: Above all, you come up against physical limitations and have to learn to live with the fact that you can't do certain things anymore. That isn't always easy.

My experience of letting go started early, with music, which has always meant so much to me throughout my entire life. I already shared with you how my cello, as "my baby," accompanied me to Sweden and then Africa. It was later joined by my viola da gamba and a spinet from Switzerland. Over the years, I had to let go of playing these instruments due to my visual impairment. It began with the cello and the viola da gamba – I couldn't read the music any more. For a while, I tried to overcome this by tying a string between the cupboards in my Elim living room and hanging sheet music from it. But once I had the notes close enough to my eyes to read them, I couldn't see my instrument down below. It gets extremely tricky when you can only feel around on the fingerboard of your instrument, without being able to see it. It made me very sad. I always loved to play, but I was really bad at playing from memory. Even as a student I had struggled with that, and my cello teacher told me that I had no kinaesthetic memory in my finger muscles.

I haven't played since those days in Elim. I passed on the cello to the youngest daughter of my colleague Carel IJsselmuiden. At the moment of giving it away, I realised that I was losing an important part of myself. What remains is my joy in listening to music. For a while, I had a subscription in Basel for tickets for chamber music and symphony concerts, but that too is over. I no longer like going out in the evenings – it has become a real chore, since I get tired so quickly. The things I enjoy most now are Sunday afternoon concerts in Basel's churches.

Closely associated with my visual impairment is also my declining hearing. I have a hard time following table talk, unless someone sitting beside me continually explains what's being discussed. But few people have that level of sensitivity. Oral presentations often rush past me like a waterfall, especially those of younger people, who often speak quickly and without careful articulation. It's the same thing in the theatre. These actors today? Either they shout, or they whisper, or they turn their backs to you – I scarcely understand anything. But instead of getting upset about it, I just avoid going now.

Slips of the tongue and the loss of short-term memory would be another whole discussion, but I don't worry about those things a bit, because I know they are totally normal. I'm always able to laugh about it…

G: But you have a fabulous long-term memory, as this biography demonstrates!

E: Yes, I know. People's long-term memory usually stays intact until the very end. In addition to everything else, I've become slower in everything I do. I need a lot more time to perform all the tasks of a normal day, and I often get frustrated when I can't keep up with my daily schedule. Many things get left undone and pile up. It's especially hard for me when I fail to keep in touch with old friends and acquaintances, and they wind up feeling neglected. My circle of friends now includes some younger people, and my interests have changed a bit. You have to choose what's important now. On the whole, however, I think I'm very good at letting go of things and saying goodbye. Our little vacation home in Ticino, for instance, was a real source of connection with my brother Ernst. I can still picture him there in the garden tending to his roses, surrounded by the Ticino countryside he loved. When I said farewell to the place, I did a lot of sketching for one last time. I tried to look at everything through his eyes once more. And then I could "turn the page". This was important to me.

I also had to say goodbye to long mountain hikes, and learn to be happy taking walks using a walking stick, as I did again recently in Splügen. I still remember the wonderful, high mountain hike with you through the Fuorn Pass to Lü three years ago, in the autumn. I know I can't do that any more. It took us five hours, of course, rather than the three written on the yellow signposts, but it was lovely to experience the Arvenwald, the forest of Swiss pines *(Pinus cembra)* once more; to walk along narrow paths and look at the late-flowering plants, the trees beginning to take on their autumn colours, the sunshine, and the mountain peaks fresh with snow.

Finally, ageing also means saying goodbye to a growing number of my friends and contemporaries. People react very differently. One of them was constantly complaining about what she could no longer do, while another, lying in hospital with cancer, had such a positive attitude, being thankful for all that the nurses did for her, that it made me happy, too. Most recently, I lost my dear school friend, Irène Bourcart, who meant so much to me when we met again in Africa. I was still able to keep her company in the old people's home, when she was very sick with Alzheimer's disease. Whenever I spoke about the time in Africa, she would perk up, and she even began speaking fluent Tsonga again on one occasion when Selina came to visit with me. Once – she was still able to speak a little – she expressed her wish to go skiing once more in the mountains. I took up the theme and planned the holiday with her and described how it would be. It made her happy. I remain friends with her sister Noémi who also means a lot to me, though we seldom get to see each other.

G: What joys remain for you?

E: I'm thankful for everything I can still do. I can walk steadily, and go for short strolls and little hikes. I like being at home more and having time to enjoy my balcony garden, the little green wilderness. Especially dear to me is the moment at dusk when I sit in my comfortable chair in front of the little greenhouse, maybe read a short text or just quietly relax, gaze at the bamboo swaying in the breeze, and let my thoughts wander into the green countryside. If there's something to admire on the balcony, I fetch my neighbour Annegreth, or she might fetch me to her balcony, to gaze with her at whatever is in bloom. She is also a passionate gardener, and has offered to help me with weeding. I have a lot of fun playing patience, or playing Scrabble with Gaby, and of course I enjoy having theological discussions with my friend Marianne Graf. On Sundays, I've found a good way to structure my day by going to worship at St Paul's church, and staying afterwards to drink coffee. It gives me a chance to be around a good community and meet new people.

For the same reason, to enjoy the company of others, I've organised an individual weekly schedule for my midday meals. I don't have the energy to cook every day any more, but I absolutely don't want to have the meals delivered by the "Meals on Wheels" service. Then I'd just be sitting alone in front of my plate yet again! So on Tuesdays I go to the lunch for elderly people served in the Church Hall, where I see people I wouldn't meet otherwise. My friend Marie-Claire Barth invites me to lunch once a week, and other friends are very hospitable too. But two or three times in between, and every evening, I enjoy cooking something for myself.

Once a year, I bake a big cherry cake (a "Kirsipfann"), which lands in the freezer and is eventually eaten in the pleasant company of my neighbours. There's a real sense of community in our building, where six of the 12 flats are occupied by single women. Getting together to eat my cherry cake has become a tradition. And I know that if I'm not doing well, there are caring people around me. Isn't it wonderful to live like this?

I'd like to have a little more time – after the big effort of this book – to make a cosy clutter out of the big jumble of stuff I currently have. That will be enough for me. Having some time to read would be nice, too. In the past, I had to make time to read in bed at night, since there was so much going on during the day. But my eyes are no longer good enough. So now I enjoy times when good friends offer to read aloud to me, and interesting radio programmes.

G: The last question is your own: Why am I still here?

E: Perhaps thanks to my guardian angel? I have certainly been spared many times when things could have gone badly. I've often put my guardian angel to the test, and so far he hasn't failed me. It started when I was a baby. One day, my pushchair took off by itself when it had been parked in front of a shop, and rolled down a steep road with me in it, before tipping over. Nothing happened to me at all!

I have a habit of focusing so fully on one thing in particular that I become oblivious to the dangers around me. Once, a doctor colleague saved me in the nick of time from being attacked and strangled by an Indian mental patient, when I had become mesmerised by a bug on her sari while examining her. Another time, I had collected a visitor at the station in Louis-Trichardt, and popped into the station café to buy bread. I was all ready to pay, when I was suddenly grabbed from behind by Silas, our driver, and pulled out of the way of a group of thieves who had crowded round me and were about to grab my purse. If that wasn't my guardian angel!

But the angel's master-stroke happened on Pisanghoek, a mountain range between Louis Trichardt and Zimbabwe. I went there on an excursion with Rev. Wilhelm Vischer and his wife from Basel. As we drove, Wilhelm and I were singing the 23rd Psalm in two parts, according to my sister Trudi's very lovely setting, whose creation we had all been involved in. I didn't have a driver's license yet, but sat at the wheel on the steep zigzag route. Right beside the curving road, the terrain abruptly fell off into a deep ravine. Suddenly someone yelled behind me: "Stop, stop!" I had come within an inch of missing a hairpin bend as we sang. All of us would have plunged into the ravine. I still get gooseflesh thinking about it. And in 2008, my guardian angel was put to work again when he rescued me from three life-threatening situations in a row. First of all, I fell asleep while reading and a corner of my pillow had already begun to give off smoke when it came too close to my bedside lamp, but I woke up just in time. Then I had a fall on the stairs at the entrance to my home, where a passer by helped me to my feet unharmed. The third incident was a sudden increase in blood pressure. It was over 230 – but I was able to receive medical attention just in time. The reason for it was a shocking telephone call from Selina, in which she told me that the Care Groups were dying out. Luckily, a good solution was eventually found, and the Care Groups have been strengthened with Selina's help.

After so many rescues, I have to ask myself: What is the reason I'm still here, at my advanced age? Only God can answer that. But maybe I shall find some clues?

One thing that I am thankful for is that I have not lost the capacity to marvel at things! This ability to wonder, and be amazed, is something that one can't take for granted. These days, I feel that more and more people have lost it. In a little book by Kurt Marti, one can read these lines:

"Do miracles exist? Yes. You, for example. Me too, I suppose. And life in general; every living thing."[3]

Seeing the summit of Mount Kilimanjaro was just such a miracle for me, during a trip to a game reserve in southern Kenya. Its snow-capped peak is usually shrouded by a veil of cloud. When I got up at six in the morning to go for a walk, the clouds suddenly parted, and the mountain peak was revealed for just a moment. It was overwhelming. I took a photo, thinking at the same time: "You don't have the right to capture this sacred moment in a picture. It's almost a sacrilege." It was a great moment of wonder for me.

Indeed: Every living thing is a reason for marvelling over and over again – everything that I have a chance to discover on walks and in my balcony garden. My beloved *Oenothera odorata*, for example, when it finally blooms in the evening, for a single night. In early summer, it might produce five, six, or even more blossoms all at once. Then I call Annegreth over and we watch as the petals open and unfold to form perfect cup shaped flowers, which are gone by the morning. We inhale its special fragrance and know that it's a plant with diverse gifts. It is beautiful, healing, and edible – you could even scatter its petals over a salad, but they're far too precious for that. That would be sacrilege for me, and I wouldn't do it. For me, the *Oenothera* symbolises a life as it should be. I've tried to put it into words:

OENOTHERA ODORATA

In the evening
When your blossoms
Unfold into
A perfect cup
My heart cries out in amazement
That's how I would like to be
Aglow in the darkness
Opening up
To receive and to give
Healing and pure
Freed and setting free

But reason warns
Not yet
Unless
For a moment
When a waft
Of the divine mystery
Touches me softly
In passing
And
So I hope
One day
To be seen
As God meant me to be[4]

Endnotes

1. A Swiss politician, teacher and writer, very active on behalf of Human Rights. One of his mandates was as UN Special Rapporteur on the right to food, from 2000 to 2008.
2. This international organisation was founded in 1908 by Rev. Ernst Christoffel to work for the blind. In German the name "Cristoffel Blindenmission" is still in use. In English, the organisation is now called Christian Blind Mission, or simply CBM. It is a Christian humanitarian organization aiming to improve the lives of people with various disabilities.
3. Kurt Marti. *Von der Weltleidenschaft Gottes* (On God's Passion for the World). Radius Verlag GmbH, Stuttgart 1997
4. The last line of the poem is a reference to I Corinthians 13, verse 12, "… then shall I know even as also I am known" (King James Version).

Erika's favourite flower,
Oenothera odorata

Illustrations

All photographs stem from Erika Sutter's private collection. Exceptions are listed in the following. To the extent known, the names of the photographers are provided.

Frontispiece: Gertrud Stiehle: Private Collection Gertrud Stiehle.

Immersing myself in the life of Erika Sutter
Erika and Gertrud: Photographer Frances Lund.

Chapter VI
Erika operating (p. 50): Photographer Hans Sutter.
Measles in malnourished children (p. 57): Photographer Leslie Lawson.
Erika with Ilse and C.F. Beyers Naudé (p. 64): Photographer Pauline Bill.

Chapter VII
Erika with the first two Care Group motivators (p. 78): Photographer Rob Collins.
Care Group motivator Florence (p. 80): Photographer Leslie Lawson.
Dancing Care Group (p. 88): Photographer M.A. Gneist.
Selina, Erika and Frances (p. 93): Photographer Gaby Sutter.

Chapter VIII
Farewell from the Care Groups at Giyani (p. 95): Photographer Lennard Karlsson.
Erika waves Goodbye (p. 96): Photographer Lennard Karlsson.
Soglio (p. 101): Photographer Getrud Lukanow.
Erika with her brother Ernst (p. 110): Photographer Frances Lund.

Bibliography

List of publications by Erika Sutter
(in chronological order)

Sutter E. – Blindness among South African Negroes in the Far Northern Transvaal. *S.A. Arch. Ophthal.*, 1973, 1, 105–115.

Ballard R.C., Sutter E.E., and Fotheringham P. – Trachoma in a rural South African community. *Am. J. Trop. Med. Hyg.*, 1978, 27, 113–120.

Sutter E. and Ballard R.C. – A Community Approach to Trachoma Control in the Northern Transvaal. *S.A. med. J.*, 1978, 53, 622–625.

Sutter E. – The Care Groups: a community involvement in Primary Health Care. SALDRU/SAMST, *Economics of Health in South Africa*, U.C.T., Ravan Press, Johannesburg, 1979, 293–302.

Abrahams C., Ballard R.C. and Sutter E., – The Pathology of Trachoma in a Black South African Population. *S.Afr. med. J.*, 1979, 55, 1115–1118.

Ballard R.C., Fehler H.G., Baerveldt G, Owen G., Sutter E. and Mphahlele M. – The epidemiology and geographical distribution of trachoma in Lebowa. *S.Afr. med. J.*, 1981, 60, 531–535.

Niederer W., Sutter E. – Das Oberlidentropion und dessen differenzierte Behandlung. *Klin. Mbl.Augenheilk.*, 1981, 17, 8, 464-468.

Sutter E. – *Mahlo, Mahungu ya Nyanisi Rikhotso*. Sasavona Books, Braamfontein, South Africa, 1981.

Sutter E. – Community participation in the prevention of disability. *Rehabilitation in S.A.*, 1982, 26, 65–70.

Sutter E. and Ballard R.C. – Community participation in the control of Trachoma in Gazankulu. *Soc. Sci. Med.*, 1983, 17, 1813–1817.

Sutter E. – Training of eye care workers and their integration in Gazankulu's comprehensive health services. *Soc. Sci.Med.* 1983, 17, 1809–1812.

Ballard R.C., Fehler H.G., Fotheringham P., Sutter E. & Treharne J.D. – Trachoma in South Africa. *Soc. Sci. Med.* 1983, 17, 1755–1765.

Sutter E. – Wird Nyanisi erblinden? *KEM, Kollektenverein der Basler Mission*, 1988, 7–10.

Sutter E., Foster A. and Francis V. – *Hanyane, A Village Struggles for Eye Health*. Macmillan Publishers, London, 1989. ISBN 0-333-51092-5.

French edition: *Hanyane, - Bien voire et mieux vivre au village*. 1993, International Centre for Eye Health, London.

Sutter E. – Vom Operationssaal zum Gemüsegarten (I). *Bulletin medicus mundi Schweiz*, 1990, 42, 13–31.

Sutter E. – Vom Operationssaal zum Gemüsegarten (II). *Bulletin medicus mundi Schweiz*, 1990, 43, 13–20.

Sutter E. – Primary Health Care at the Margins. *Critical Health*, 1991, 36/37, 14–23.

Sutter E. – Das Trachom, eine Seuche der Armen in der Dritten Welt. *Bulletin medicus mundi Schweiz*, 1992, 49/50, 21–30.

Sutter E. – Trachoma, a disease of poverty in developing countries. *Bulletin medicus mundi Schweiz*, 1995, 56, 26–36.

Sutter E. and Maphorogo S. – Integration of community-based trachoma control in primary health care in South Africa – Intégration du controle du trachome dans les communautés villageoises, au sein des soins de santé primaire en Afrique du Sud. *Rev. Internat. Trachome*, 1996 French: 17–29, English: 31–48.

Sutter E. and Maphorogo S. – The Elim Care Group Project, Women's groups as health promoters in a rural area in South Africa. *Memisa Medisch*, 1997, 63, 50–58.

Sutter E. and IJsselmuiden Carel – Still going after all these years...?! *Bulletin medicus mundi*, 1998, Nr. 69, 1–15.

Sutter E. – Frauen wollen leben, Care Groups in Südafrika. *Soziale Medizin*, 2000, Nr. 6, 12–17.

Sutter E. – Wir haben unsere Füsse gefunden. *Schritte ins Offene*, 1999, 3, 3–6.

French edition: Quand le fortuit devient engagement. *Perspectives missionnaires*, 2001/1 Nr 41.

Sutter E. – The Elim Care Groups: A Community Project for the Control of Trachoma. *Community Eye Health*, 2001, 14, 47–49.

Maphorogo S., Sutter E. and Jenkins J. – *The Community is my University, A voice from the grass roots on rural health and development*. KIT Publishers Royal Tropical Institute, Amsterdam, 2003. On CD TALC, St. Albans, UK, www.talcuk.org, 2009.

Further publications on the Care Groups:

Tollman S. et al. – Evaluation of a community approach to preventable disease in Gazankulu. SALDRU/SAMST, *Economics of health in South Africa*, UCT., 1979, 303–317. Ravan Press, Johannesburg.

Karlsson E.L. – Care groups and primary health care in rural areas. *Israel. J. Med. Sci.*, 1983, 19, 731–733.

Lund F.J. – *The community based approach to development: A description and analysis of three rural community health projects*. Centre for Social and Development Studies, University of Natal, Durban, 1987.

Maphorogo S. – Care Group Motivator: A Personal View. *Critical Health*, 1991, 36/37, 24–27.

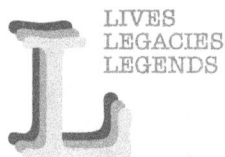

LIVES
LEGACIES
LEGENDS

4 Ursula Trüper
The Invisible Woman. Zara Schmelen. African Mission Assistant at the Cape and in Namaland (2006)

Africa in 1814: a 36-year-old German missionary exploring what is now southern Namibia marries the 20-year-old Zara, a Nama woman, whom he had baptized a few months previously. She helps him with translations and in transcribing her language into a wirtten form, bears him four children, and dies in 1831.

Those are the bare bones of a story that Ursula Trüper has fleshed out into this fascinating account about the African woman and her German husband, the missionary Johann Hinrich Schmelen. He is recognized today as a pioneer in the study of Khoekhoekowab, the Nama language. His wife Zara and her contributions, on the other hand, are rarely mentioned, let alone acknowledged. This book rectifies that neglect and makes an important contribution to the steadily growing literature on the role of African women in African history.

6 Hans Buser
In Ghana at Independence. Stories of a Swiss Salesman (2010)

The Swiss salesman, Hans Buser, experienced at close quarters the political, social and economic ups and downs of a young Ghana in the period immediately following independence. His stories and reminiscences of those turbulent years between 1956 and 1965 are characterised by sharp observation, insight and humour.

Hans Buser was born in Switzerland in 1934. In 1956 he made his first trip to Africa as an employee of the Basel Union Trading Company. He made numerous friends among his African colleagues and household staff, as well as in the circle of politicians who had led the country to independence under the leadership of President Kwame Nkrumah.

7 Israel Goldblatt
Building Bridges. Namibian Nationalists Clemens Kapuuo, Hosea Kutako, Brendan Simbwaye, Samuel Witbooi (2010)

Windhoek in the early 1960s: the 34-year-old politician Clemens Kapuuo knocks at the door of the senior advocate Israel Goldblatt to solicit advice regarding the myriad of difficulties encountered by Africans daily under the apartheid regime. An unusual relationship and friendship develops, one that transcends the racial divide in this South African-governed Territory and will last for nearly 10 years.

Israel Goldblatt's notes on meetings with politician Clemens Kapuuo, Kaptein Samuel Witbooi, Brendan Simbwaye, Chief Hosea Kutako and a group of younger nationalists, among them Rev. Bartholomews Karuaera and Levy Nganjone, were discovered after his death and form the core of this book. They are complemented by additional biographical information about his interlocutors, and annotations that place his notes in their historical and political context.

Illustrated with many photographs, this publication pays tribute to Israel Goldblatt and the Namibian nationalists who attempted to build bridges where apartheid entrenched racism and suspicion.